Elder Care

SAGE SOURCEBOOKS FOR THE HUMAN SERVICES SERIES

Series Editors: ARMAND LAUFFER and CHARLES GARVIN

Recent Volumes in this Series

Elder Care

Family Training and Support

Amanda Smith Barusch

Sage Sourcebooks for

the Human Services Series
18

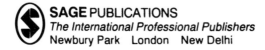
SAGE PUBLICATIONS
The International Professional Publishers
Newbury Park   London   New Delhi

10-16-95

For information address:

SAGE Publications, Inc.
2455 Teller Road
Newbury Park, California 91320

SAGE Publications Ltd.
6 Bonhill Street
London EC2A 4PU
United Kingdom

SAGE Publications India Pvt. Ltd.
M-32 Market
Greater Kailash I
New Delhi 110 048 India

Printed in the United States of America

Library of Congress Cataloging-in-Publication Data

Barusch, Amanda Smith.
    Elder care: family training and support / Amanda Smith Barusch.
        p.   cm.   — (Sage sourcebooks for the human services series;
v. 18)
    Includes bibliographical references and index.
    ISBN 0-8039-4227-3 (c). —ISBN 0-8039-4185-4 (p)
    1. Aged—Care—Study and teaching—United States. 2. Caregivers—
Training of—United States.   I. Title. II. Series.
HV1461.B35   1991
362.6—dc20   91-11225
                                                                                        CIP

FIRST PRINTING, 1991

Sage Production Editor: Diane S. Foster

CONTENTS

ACKNOWLEDGMENTS

Elder care and the *Wellsprings* training curriculum represent the combined efforts of many. A few can be mentioned here. The staff of the University of Utah's Caregiver Support Project contributed brilliance, enthusiasm, and lots of time. The faculty of the University of Utah Graduate School of Social Work provided moral support and ready answers to dozens of questions.

David Turner and Maggie Godfrey developed and taught the original *Wellsprings* curriculum. Dana Cochran-Wiley and Joette Langianese wrote guidelines for implementing training programs that are incorporated in Chapter 2. Larry Barusch and Steve Jennings taught me about legal issues and reviewed Chapter 7. Betsy Beisecker helped me learn about talking to doctors and reviewed Chapter 8, offering wonderful suggestions. Kathleen Braza taught me about grief and offered excellent suggestions on Chapter 9. Kenneth Bender provided a helpful review of the medication management section. Elizabeth Murray contributed her infectious good humor, incredible persistence, and lots of work to research and preparation. Phyllis Barusch reviewed draft after draft, giving suggestions, corrections, and support. Vickie Schmall reviewed the manuscript, improving it substantially.

Larry, Nathan, and Ariana Barusch tolerated my unavailability with good grace, offering respite, encouragement, and reasons for delight.

The hundreds of caregivers who participated in the University of Utah's Caregiver Support Project shared their joys, tears, victories, and frustrations, providing inspiration and direction for this work. They are my *Wellsprings*, and this book is dedicated to them.

PREFACE

Caregiving combines the powerful emotions of caring with the act of giving. It is one of the finest gifts we can give to a loved one. It is also one of the most draining experiences we can face. Many family members jeopardize their ability to care for a loved one by ignoring their own needs. In so doing, they endanger their physical and emotional health. The self-love that enables caregivers to care for themselves is a vital resource, a *wellspring* that can yield innumerable benefits. This book is designed to support and encourage expressions of self-love.

A *wellspring* is a source of continual renewal. This book provides skills and knowledge that will become *wellsprings* for the caregiver. In the following pages, you will find background information designed to improve your understanding of specific problems that confront the family caregiver, as well as exercises designed to improve coping skills and interpersonal communication within the caregiving context. You also will find guidelines for designing, implementing, and evaluating a caregiver support program that includes both training and peer support. The *Wellsprings* curriculum presented here was designed by the University of Utah's Caregiver Support Project. The project is described in Appendix A.

USING THIS BOOK

The book is divided into two parts. Part I offers detailed guidelines for those interested in establishing a short-term training program for family caregivers. Part II presents background material and exercises that can be used either by trainers or by those personally involved in caregiving.

Part I includes Chapters 1 through 3. Chapter 1 introduces a framework for understanding the dynamics of a caregiving situation. Chapter 2 offers practical insights for designing and implementing caregiver support programs. Chapter 3 discusses methods for evaluating caregiver programs.

Part II, Chapters 4 through 9, includes content that can be used for training sessions or by those involved in caregiving. Chapter 4 discusses normal aging, contrasting normal age-related changes with the effects of disease. Chapter 5 addresses the emotional needs that must be met to maintain healthy family relationships. Chapter 6 describes the services and resources available in most communities, including health and social service professionals. Chapter 7 addresses legal and financial concerns. Chapter 8 presents two caregiving skills: managing medications and ensuring home safety. Chapter 9 discusses grief and dying. A list of resources is provided at the end of each chapter, as well as suggestions for trainers.

Appendix A provides background on the evaluation of the University of Utah's Caregiver Support Project. Training exercises are presented in Appendix B, and Appendix C includes a list of books and organizations.

INTRODUCTION: Long-Term Care of America's Frail Elderly

Simple demographics have brought the care of older adults to the status of a major national concern. The 1970s saw a 32% increase in the number of Americans aged 75 and over (U.S. Bureau of Census, 1989). Similarly, the number of Americans 85 and older increased by 165% from 1960 to 1982 (U.S. Senate Special Committee on Aging, 1986). This growth is projected to accelerate until 2050, when 37,039,000 Americans join the ranks of the "old-old" (U.S. Bureau of Census, 1982). Because advanced age leads to an increased risk of chronic illness, this "abundance of life" brings with it overwhelming demands for institutions and individuals concerned with caring for elderly who become sick or disabled.

Most of these demands reflect the rising incidence of chronic disabilities that require "long-term care." Long-term care is a catchall term, referring to the array of medical, personal, and social services available to meet the needs of the chronically impaired. Until recently, the term referred primarily to the 24-hour care provided in a nursing home. As a result of growing interest in alternatives to institutional care, as well as increased recognition of the family's involvement in care, this definition has expanded to include a broad range or a continuum of alternatives. This continuum ranges from home care provided entirely by family members to institutional care with no family involvement. Caregivers and the professionals who serve them need to be aware of the diverse options available for providing satisfactory long-term care.

Several distinct groups provide long-term care to America's frail elderly. They include family caregivers, health care professionals, and social service providers. Further, long-term care can be provided in a variety of settings, including private homes, adult day care centers, supportive residential facilities, and nursing homes.

LONG-TERM CARE PROVIDERS

Many individuals provide long-term care. The needs of any individual will be met by a unique constellation involving some or all of these.

Family Caregivers

The tremendous contribution of family members to the long-term care of the elderly is reflected in the widely quoted estimate offered by the National Center for Health Statistics. Based on 268,000 household interviews conducted between 1966 and 1968, it is estimated that 80% of the home health care received by the elderly in this country was provided by family members (National Center for Health Statistics, 1972).

Who are the caregivers? Stone, Cafferata, and Sangl (1987) studied 6,393 caregivers, using a nationwide sample that is representative of family members who provide care. They report that those who care for the frail elderly are primarily women (72%), with adult daughters making up 29%, wives 32%, and husbands 13% of caregivers. One third of caregivers surveyed were the sole source of assistance, and most of these sole caregivers were spouses. Daughters were much more likely than sons to be the primary or sole provider of care. Most (three fourths) of the caregivers lived with the care receivers. A significant minority (almost one third) were poor or near poor, and one third reported their health was fair or poor. Chapter 1 offers an ecological approach to assessing the dynamics of family caregiving.

Health Care Professionals

After family members, nurses emerge as the major providers of home care. The National Center for Health Statistics (1972) reported that 10% of those receiving home care had some care provided by a nurse. Other health care professionals typically involved in long-term care include physicians, rehabilitation specialists, and pharmacists.

Chapter 8 presents descriptions of the contributions of these specialists to long-term care, as well as suggestions for choosing and working effectively with a physician. Chapter 9 presents information on financing long-term care through Medicare and Medicaid.

Social Service Providers

The availability of social services for the elderly varies widely from community to community. What uniformity does exist results largely from the system established under the Older Americans Act of 1965. This legislation created a network of agencies called Area Agencies on Aging (AAAs) that covers the United States and its territories. AAAs must provide services that help people get access to other needed services (transportation, outreach, and information and referral), in-home services (homemaker and home health aides, visiting and telephone reassurance, and chore maintenance), and legal services. Other services that may be provided include senior centers, meals on wheels, case management, health screening, senior companions, and volunteer opportunities. Often social services of this kind will help maintain an older person at home despite illness and disability. Chapter 6 describes these services and issues involved in accessing them, and Chapter 8 discusses financing available through Medicare and Medicaid.

LONG-TERM CARE SETTINGS

The choice of a setting in which to provide care for a frail family member is an emotional and confusing issue. The goal of caregiver interventions should not be to support one setting to the exclusion of others (e.g., to keep patients at home) but to support the choice of an appropriate setting for the individual and the family.

Private Homes

The vast majority of long-term care takes place in private homes. For the patient, home care can have several advantages: Familiar surroundings require fewer adjustments and so produce less confusion and disorientation; the home environment allows for visits and assistance from family and friends in an informal atmosphere; home care often optimizes patient control, with a minimum of regulatory intervention and professional authorities; and finally, home care is consistent with the need for privacy that is keenly felt by many older Americans.

Caregivers, too, tend to prefer home care. Most believe that the quality of care available at home exceeds that in other settings. Policymakers prefer home care as it does not usually entail large public expenditures.

But long-term care in private homes has several disadvantages, among them the high cost born by family caregivers (see Chapter 2); the risk of accidents and injury in homes that do not accommodate the patient's disabilities (see Chapter 9); and the possibility of inadequate care, when family caregivers lack the skills necessary to meet the medical needs of the patient. There is also the growing concern that abuse and neglect of frail elders often goes undetected in private homes.

Clearly some individuals cannot receive care at home. These are elderly without support systems in or around their homes, those whose needs (medical and otherwise) exceed the capacities of available caregivers, and those whose behavior represents a threat to themselves or others at home.

Adult Day Care Centers

Adult day care was introduced in the United States in the 1960s, as a program of training and recreation for hospitalized elderly. Since then adult day care has evolved and expanded. Now it is primarily used to support impaired adults living in the community. Using either a social or a medical model, programs offer daily care. Tate and Brennan (1988) documented the rapid expansion of adult day care, reporting that there were only 20 such facilities in the 1970s, and well over 1,200 by 1980. The availability of adult day care varies widely throughout the country, with programs clustered in metropolitan areas. It is seldom available to those living in rural areas.

Supportive Residential Facilities

When an older person's home is no longer suitable, either because of isolated location, size, or obstacles such as stairs, independent living may still be an alternative. Housing units specifically designed for the elderly offer minimal care and maintenance requirements, and often provide opportunities for socializing. Those who require daily care or supervision may find that board and care homes, adult foster care, or sheltered care are workable alternatives. Unfortunately, availability of these options is often limited and in many states these facilities are not licensed or regulated. Where there is no licensing, the quality of care provided can vary widely.

Nursing Homes

Despite the stigma attached to institutional care, nursing homes provide a vital contribution to the long-term care of America's elderly. At any given time, only 5 to 6% of those over 65 live in a nursing home (Palmore, 1976; U.S. Bureau of the Census, 1976). But the chances that a person will require institutional care increase exponentially with age. For example, using nationwide data, Liang and Tu (1986) estimated that Americans over 85 would spend 4.3 of their remaining 6.1 years (or 70% of their average life expectancy) in a nursing home. This compares to 23% for those over 65, and 5% for those under 45 years of age.

There are about 16,000 nursing homes in the United States, concentrated for the most part in urban areas (Sirrocco, 1989). They range from "clean, cheerful homes where the patients are well cared for and comfortable" to "smelly warehouses where patients are neglected and overdrugged to keep them quiet" (Alzheimer's Disease Research, 1987).

The choice to use a nursing home is extremely difficult for caregivers and other family members. By providing a forum for objective discussion of this alternative, caregiver groups can help ensure appropriate use of this important long-term care resource and ease the pain experienced by many families. Chapter 6 provides more information on placement as a care option.

Part I

DESIGNING, IMPLEMENTING, AND EVALUATING A CAREGIVER SUPPORT PROGRAM

This part of the *Wellsprings* curriculum is primarily designed for those interested in developing caregiver support programs. The programs now provided throughout the country typically use one of two models. The first is a "support group" format. In this model the primary purpose of the program is to offer peer support and exchange experiences. Information may be presented, but training is not a primary goal. Often support groups are ongoing, with members joining and leaving as their personal needs dictate. In the second, the "training" format, the primary purpose is to provide caregivers the skills and knowledge necessary to better care for themselves and their loved ones. Peer support may be a secondary objective. Usually training programs are offered for a limited period, with all members beginning at the same time. One advantage of the training model is that caregivers are usually more willing to participate in educational programs than in support groups. The *Wellsprings* program is primarily a training program. Sessions are organized around specific information and skills. Peer support is optimized through the use of exercises and structured discussion of personal experiences. The program might be used to enhance an ongoing support group, as part of a long-term training package, or as an independent short-term training effort.

Part I of this volume includes four chapters. Chapter 1 uses an ecological framework to present background material for use in assessing the family caregiving situation. Chapter 2 offers practical advice on designing and implementing a program. Recruiting, screening, scheduling, transportation, respite care, and interpersonal dynamics are discussed, as well as the unique concerns of four special groups: rural

1

caregivers, men, ethnic minorities, and isolated caregivers. Chapter 3 describes evaluation designs ranging from simple to elaborate, as well as specific measures for use in outcome evaluation.

Chapter 1

AN ECOLOGICAL FRAMEWORK
FOR ASSESSMENT: *Resources*
and Constraints

Each provider who interacts with a caregiver is involved to some extent in assessment. This might be as simple as a gut-level message saying, "This woman is *desperate* for help," or as complex as a 2-hour interview based on a structured protocol. This chapter is designed not to replace existing assessment practices but to strengthen them. The discussion is based on a conceptual framework, derived from an ecological perspective. This framework directs attention to the wide range of resources available to the caregiver, as well as the competing pressures and demands on caregivers and others involved. The patient is considered an active participant in care and an important determinant of caregiver well-being. The personal experience of caregiving is considered—the factors that contribute to a decision to assume the role, and the personal consequences of that decision. The rewards of caregiving as well as the strains are reviewed with a view toward facilitating empathetic intervention. This chapter also discusses the unique aspects of caregiving done by husbands, wives, daughters, and other family members. Certain dynamics are typical of each caregiving configuration, and it may be helpful to identify the special needs of each family member.

THE ECOLOGICAL FRAMEWORK

By directing attention to the context of the caregiving situation, an ecological perspective encourages holistic assessment. Service providers tend to focus on an identified client to the exclusion of other people involved. This applies as much to human service professionals as it does to medical professionals. Medical professionals may overlook the needs and concerns of caregivers as they focus on the health needs of care receivers. Similarly, those who are primarily concerned with supporting caregivers tend to ignore the patient, or treat him or her as an object rather than an active participant in the caregiving situation. Use of an ecological perspective will help overcome this tendency.

With its roots in evolutionary biology, the ecological perspective directs attention to the interaction between a person and the environment (Bronfenbrenner, 1979). The ecosystem of caregiver and care receiver can be characterized as having both elements and processes. The elements are the people involved: the caregiver, care receiver, other family members, friends and neighbors, professional service providers, and policymakers (see Figure 1.1). These people can serve as resources in support of the caregiver or as constraints, limiting the number of options available. Often the same person does both. From an ecological perspective, adaptation is a central process in the caregiving situation. Adaptation is discussed in the closing section of this chapter.

PEOPLE IN THE CAREGIVING ECOSYSTEM

The Caregiver

Careful assessment of a caregiver will address the meaning he or she assigns to the role as well as the costs and rewards experienced. The caregiver has chosen to assume an extremely demanding role at high personal cost. Living the "36-hour day" described by Mace and Rabins (1981), the caregiver is likely to experience exhaustion, loss of privacy, fear, embarrassment, anxiety, grief, daily irritations, loss of freedom, financial deprivation, social isolation, worry, and guilt (Archbold, 1982; Cantor, 1983; Robinson & Thurnher, 1979).

Fengler and Goodrich (1979) were among the first writers to acknowledge the strain involved in caregiving. They interviewed 15

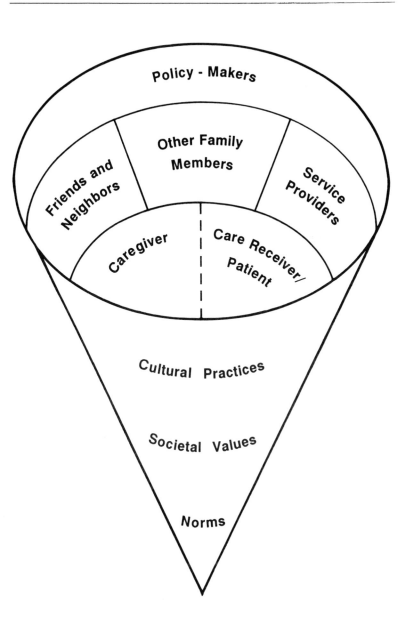

Figure 1.1 The Caregiving Ecosystem: Individuals in an Expanding Social Context

wives of disabled men and found that they had low morale. The authors noted that adequate income, contact with family and friends, companionship with spouse, and the ability to leave home for errands contributed to higher morale among these spouse caregivers. Fengler and Goodrich described caregiving spouses as "hidden patients" and recommended that services be established to help them in their role. Since then, researchers have continued to document the high cost associated with caregiving.

Given the high cost of caregiving, why would a rational person ever assume the role? Cicirelli addressed this question in his 1981 book on the role of adult children in helping elderly parents. He interviewed members of both generations to identify factors that sustain or activate helping behavior by adult children. Factors considered included attachment, filial obligation, interpersonal conflict, and parent dependency. His analysis suggested that a central factor that sustained helping was attachment, "an emotional or affectional bond between two people" (p. 19)—in other words, love.

His findings were echoed in responses of caregivers who participated in the University of Utah's Caregiver Support Project (CSP): "We enjoy being together, I love him very much" (55-year-old wife). "Because I love him" (57-year-old wife). "Our lives are intertwined around each other" (75-year-old husband).

Caregivers also mentioned the lack of acceptable alternatives. Given the high cost of nursing home care, and their aversion to placing a loved one in such a setting, they felt they had no choice: "I didn't know anything else to do" (62-year-old wife). "We are a team and I don't like nursing homes" (81-year-old husband). "I knew I could give her more attention than she would ever get in a nursing home" (87-year-old husband).

The meaning a caregiver assigns to the role will be heavily influenced by his or her primary motivation. In my observation, caregivers who were primarily motivated by an aversion to nursing home care (those who felt they had no acceptable alternative) experienced considerably more stress and less growth in the role than those who described love or concern as their primary motivation.

Caregivers who are motivated by love and concern may have better access to the rewards of caregiving. These are less well documented than the costs, but Robinson and Thurnher (1979) reported that caregivers appreciated the opportunities for close contact with a loved one; the chance to reminisce with a spouse, or learn about family history from an aged parent. Similarly, Kinney and Stephens (1989) reported that the "uplifts" of caregiving related to the wellbeing of the patient. These uplifts were more available to the more intensely involved caregiver.

The caregiver role also offers control. The illness of a spouse or parent can provide the caregiver a long-awaited opportunity to "take charge" of the patient's life. But control is a double-edged sword. It brings with it potentially overwhelming responsibility. Thus the caregiver who has a lifelong habit of assuming responsibility may find him- or herself overwhelmed by guilt or, worse, depression. Krause (1986) reported that the "inner locus of control" is associated with higher rates of depression. He suggested that people who generally assume control of events tend to blame themselves, even when faced with the uncontrollable stresses brought on by old age. Other researchers have described the same relationship between high self-efficacy or inner locus of control and depression and failure to cope (Pagel, Becker, & Coppel, 1985; West & Simons, 1983).

Caregivers are needed. Whether care receivers acknowledge their dependency or not, the fact of being indispensable can be a source of satisfaction. It also can be a source of terror. A primary concern of caregivers in CSP was fear that their own health would deteriorate (Barusch, 1988). One effective slide show on caregiving, "The Dollmaker," depicts a situation in which a caregiver dies before the patient. This show taps into a fear that can motivate caregivers to focus on their well-being. ("The Dollmaker" is available through Oregon State University Extension Service; see Resources section, Chapter 6).

Ethyl Shanas (1979) identified what she termed the "principle of substitution," which determines who will help an older person who becomes ill. In essence, she suggests that older people rely primarily on close relatives, the spouse and children. They will then substitute more remote kin when these family members are not available. This hierarchy will determine to whom an older person turns for assistance. The response of potential caregivers will depend on resources and competing demands.

Spouse Caregivers:
Unique Concerns and Opportunities

The spouse serves for many (particularly men) as the first line of defense against some functional losses of old age. Only one out of every three older women is married and living with her husband, but most older men have access to a spouse for assistance (Shanas, 1980).

The intimacy of the marital relationship presents both problems and opportunities for spouse caregivers. Caring for a disabled spouse has been described as a "long good-bye." This illustrates a primary difficulty that spouse caregivers confront: anticipatory grief. Facing the prospect of widowhood on a daily basis compounds the exhaustion brought on by caregiving. For many this means facing the loss of a lifelong companion and a central role (that of husband or wife).

Caregiving also introduces pressure to learn new skills. In marriages with traditional division of labor the caregiving wife may have to learn to manage finances, make household repairs, do lawn care, and care for automobiles. Similarly, a caregiving husband may have to learn to shop, prepare food, care for clothing, and clean house. One CSP caregiver commented, "I didn't sign up for this!" expressing her frustration at having to spend time and energy to master skills that never interested her. Others may find satisfaction and a sense of mastery in the same situation.

The physical demands of caregiving can be especially wearing on older spouses, themselves frail, sick, or even disabled. Sometimes those who work with spouse caregivers comment that it is difficult to tell who is caring for whom! Spouse caregivers often fear that their health will fail, leaving them unable to provide care.

On the other hand, the marital relationship presents opportunities to optimize the rewards in the caregiving experience. Shared reminiscence can be an especially powerful tool for relieving the tedium of caregiving, just as humor based on a lifetime of experience can offer moments of relief.

Adult Children as Caregivers:
Unique Concerns and Opportunities

Today, over 80% of the elderly have living children (Shanas, 1980). Only about 18% of those over 65 years old live in the same house with one of their children (Shanas, 1980). But many live in close proximity, yielding "intimacy at a distance," as some describe the relations of elderly with their children (Sussman, 1955). These relations involve active exchanges of visits and assistance. Most (75%) of those who live near their children see them at least weekly.

They may help with babysitting or making gifts for grandchildren, and receive help with home repairs and housework (Shanas, 1980).

Adult children who care for aging parents have been described as the "sandwich generation," sandwiched between their children and their parents; or as "women in the middle," caught in the middle with forces pulling them in several directions. This captures the predominant concern of adult children who serve as caregivers: competing demands. These may involve child-rearing responsibilities, or the daily demands of a full-time job. About one fourth of caregiving children have children under 18. Further, 44% of caregiving daughters and 55% of caregiving sons are employed (Stone et al., 1987). Other demands may come from children in college or from the caregiver's spouse. This is particularly so if other family members do not support the decision to provide care. As primary caregivers, adult children perform a delicate juggling act, trying to keep several balls in the air at once. The cost of dropping any one may be tremendous.

Like caregiving spouses, adult children experience grief. A parent's deteriorating condition brings them closer to a sense of orphanhood. Unlike spouses, adult children are genetically linked to the care receiver. If a disease has a significant genetic component, children may experience anxiety, wondering whether they see their future in their parent's disability.

Adult children also experience the discrepancy between their family roles and their caregiving responsibilities. In this society the role of child brings with it the expectation that you will respect or obey your parent. This role does not change when a parent becomes dependent. Yet caregiving responsibilities may involve decision making and intimate personal care chores that are inconsistent with these role expectations. It is hard to respect your father as you change his diaper. Yet that respect may be central to maintaining a healthy relationship. This paradox confronts caregiving children every day.

Other Family Members

Grandchildren

The vast majority (94%) of elderly who have children have grandchildren (Shanas, 1980). But the role of grandchildren in caregiving is not entirely clear. They seem willing to help in caregiving. Elaine Brody (1981) surveyed 233 families in Philadelphia and found that "granddaughters felt more strongly than the middle generation (their mothers) and much more strongly than the grandmothers . . . that older people could expect help from their grandchildren. More than three fourths of the granddaughters favored such help" (p. 475). This finding has been replicated in Japan (Campbell & Brody, 1985) and in my survey of 58 families in Shanghai, China (Barusch, Zhang, Wu, Jin, and Cai, in press).

Although grandchildren are often willing to help in caregiving, their involvement will depend to some extent on the attitudes of the older generations. There may be a worldwide tendency for older family members, both parents and grandparents, to underestimate grandchildren's willingness and capacity to provide help. This may reflect a near-universal conception of childhood and youth as a time for education, play, and career development, but not for elder care. If families cling to this conception in times of illness, caregivers may deprive themselves of a valuable source of assistance.

Grandchildren themselves can benefit from participation in caregiving. Involvement in the tasks of care can be valuable learning experiences, teaching children about illness and death, both natural parts of life. Further, the experience of caring can reaffirm their importance within the family. It also can help to keep channels of communication open, enabling grandchildren to express their grief about the illness and prepare for loss of the loved one.

Siblings and Distant Relations

Distant family members can be an important resource for people who have no closer kin. Approximately 13% of people over 65 have neither spouse nor children on whom to rely (Barusch, 1987). These people turn to siblings and distant relations for assistance.

Johnson and Catalano (1981) found that the elderly who have neither spouse nor children generally rely on nieces and nephews for assistance. Involvement of nieces and nephews is probably mediated by and dependent on strong bonds between the siblings in the older generation.

The role of siblings in caregiving is ambiguous. In one survey of childless elderly, siblings were often listed as primary caregivers (Johnson & Catalano, 1981). Typically this occurred when a spouse was unavailable to provide care. Yet Lopata (1978) reported that siblings played a very small role in the support systems of widows. In fact, the widows she surveyed were more likely to report that they provided help to their siblings than to report receiving help. Functional declines experienced by siblings are likely to make them unable to meet the care needs of a disabled brother or sister, but they can be an important source of social contact (Ward, 1978).

The Care Receiver

A patient's reaction to illness will also affect the caregiving experience. The meaning of illness and expectations of the patient role vary tremendously. To some, illness represents an opportunity to get more attention. To others it means betrayal of the body that has served so well. It is a reminder of mortality, bringing with it fears of death.

Patients also differ in their approaches to seeking support. Usually, women are less likely to rely solely on a primary caregiver for support and care. Women, especially older women, actively maintain their social relationships and networks despite their illness (Westbrook & Viney, 1983) and make greater use of professional health care providers (Lorensen, 1985). To the extent that support is received from diverse sources, the strain of caregiving may be eased.

Just as caregivers grieve the slow loss of a loved one, care receivers grieve for the roles they can no longer fill and activities they will never again enjoy. Losses also include lost expectations: dreams of golden years after retirement. Before reminiscence will be enjoyable both care receiver and caregiver need to make some progress in grieving. Grief is discussed in depth in Chapter 10.

Friends and Neighbors

Friends and neighbors can be important sources of assistance and support to both caregivers and care receivers. Several authors have suggested that help from friends is superior to that received from families (Uhlenberg, 1979; Ward, 1985). This may be true for several reasons: (a) Contact with friends is more rewarding because, as Jacques Delille pointed out in the 18th century, "Fate chooses our relatives, we choose our friends." In other words, friendship, unlike family membership is voluntary. (b) Help received from friends is less laden with inequities, disappointments, and role reversals than that received from family members. (c) Friends are most often age peers, so they may have more in common with the caregivers or care receivers. They may be better able to understand and empathize.

Typically friends and neighbors do not provide long-term, intense, hands-on care. Instead, proximity makes them available for help with emergencies and minor tasks, such as occasional transportation (Litwak, 1985). They also may be a valuable source of emotional support to both caregiver and care receiver.

Professional Service Providers

Service providers who assist caregivers include health care professionals, such as physicians and rehabilitation specialists, as well as social service professionals, such as case managers and social workers. These providers are charged with serving as resources to family caregivers, but decision-making habits and organizational constraints may limit their ability to do so.

As Frankfather (1981) reported, professionals tend to offer services that are most readily available and most professionally satisfying. Further, when public funds are not available to meet certain needs, those needs tend to go unacknowledged. Even the most well-intentioned service provider may take a narrow view of the needs of family caregivers and of alternate ways of meeting those needs. Family members may be able to expand the range of alternatives by being assertive; yet they may risk alienating the service provider. Frankfather also pointed out a tendency for service providers to "minimize risk of time consuming involvement with unruly, unstable families and clients" (p. 370).

Policymakers

Policymakers' enthusiasm for family caregiving may constrain their ability to serve as resources for caregivers. Their enthusiasm is often based on the belief that family members should provide care, that it is the *right* thing to do. This is often accompanied by the belief that the government should serve as "caregiver of last resort," entering the picture only when no other alternative is available. As a result, policymakers are often reluctant to provide services that might *replace* rather than augment family care. Although there is ample research evidence that services do not substitute for family care (Barusch & Miller, 1986), this concern arises frequently when caregiver support efforts are under consideration.

Policymakers are often willing to support home care out of their concern over the growing cost of caring for the frail elderly. As budget outlays for Medicare and Medicaid go up, those holding the public purse strings long to shift the cost of care back to the family. In this context, policymakers are reluctant to commit resources to support family and community-based care unless a net saving in public expenditures will result.

So far, demonstration and research projects have failed to support the net savings argument (Barusch & Spaid, in press; Kemper, Applebaum, & Harrigan, 1987). This, coupled with a fear that government efforts will replace family responsibility, leaves legislators and administrators reluctant to spend money in support of family care.

Nonetheless, there is growing support for home health care initiatives. In November 1987, amendments to the Older Americans Act established home care demonstration programs in five states. During the 101st Congress this program was extended to 10 states, under Title III of the Public Health Services Act. This, as well as the recent passage of the Medicaid Frail Elderly Home and Community Care Act, reveals a willingness to spend money to support home care. This willingness may be the result of a (a) traditional values of family obligation—the notion that caregivers are doing the right thing; (b) a growing awareness of the tremendous personal cost of caregiving that brings an understanding of caregivers' great need for support; (c) the (probably mistaken) idea that cost savings will result; and (d) the emergence and expansion of the home health industry. Caregiver support programs can prepare participants to work with policymakers. These programs can politicize participants, teaching them that they are not alone in their pain and with their needs. Training content might also include a discussion of the concerns described in this section. When caregiving becomes less intensely demanding participants can advocate for programs and policies in support of family care.

ADAPTATION IN THE CAREGIVING ECOSYSTEM

Adaptation is the central process in the caregiving ecosystem. Essentially, it refers to the wonderful human ability to learn and change in response to changing circumstances. Bill Cosby uses the word "re-behave" to describe the way we adjust to our aging bodies. Adaptation or re-behaving is familiar to any adult in our rapidly changing society. There are two kinds of adaptation. The first and easiest is learning new

behavior. The second and hardest is changing old behavior. Care
givers, like most of us, are eager to gain new knowledge and skills
Sometimes this can be an incentive for them to participate in trainin₤
and therapeutic activities that might also change existing behavio
that is maladaptive or destructive (also known as bad habits). Mos
bad habits once served a need. The challenge for trainers is to presen
alternative ways of meeting the same need. This frees the caregiver t(
let go of the bad habit.

Caregivers need to learn new ways of meeting old needs. For exam
ple, Mrs. A was referred to the Caregiver Support Project because th(
Veterans Administration social worker thought she was on the verg(
of collapse. She was reluctant to enroll in the training program unti
she came to see it as a way of learning new things that would mak(
her a better caregiver. Later, in group discussions, she reported that ir
addition to caring for her severely demented spouse, she wa₤
maintaining an immaculate home, doing volunteer work for a loca
charity, and loaning her son money to attend school. In her case
housekeeping and charity work were seen as "bad habits." They me₄
her needs for self-esteem, but drained energy she could not afford t(
lose. The challenge for her trainer was to identify new ways of meet
ing self-esteem needs so that she could moderate her involvement ir
housekeeping and charity work.

Reframing is a marvelous approach to adaptation. This technique
also called "cognitive restructuring," involves deliberately changin₤
the meaning we ascribe to events or circumstances. It stems from Al
bert Ellis's Rational Emotive Therapy (RET) and the idea that ₳
person's conception of a situation is more important in determinin₤
his or her reaction than the situation itself. In other words, the distress
we experience can result as much from faulty ways of construin₤
events as from the events themselves. We can therefore reduce ou₨
distress by changing our "self-talk"—eliminating negative or harshly
critical self-appraisals and irrational beliefs. (See Ellis, 1975; Gold
fried, 1980; or Meichenbaum & Jaremko, 1983, for more detailed pre
sentations of this approach.)

In Mrs. A's case, reframing was used to change the meaning she as
cribed to a disordered house. Her original interpretation was "the
woman in this home must be lazy." We asked, "Is this interpretation
realistic?" "Is it kind?" When it did not pass those tests, reframing
was introduced. Through conscious reframing her interpretation was
changed to "the woman in this home must be busy." Reframing is ₳

disarmingly simple way of changing the emotional tone of a situation. Like any new skill, it requires practice and persistence.

To adapt is to bend, like the proverbial bamboo shoot in the wind. Flexibility is a prerequisite, and caregivers vary in the extent of their flexibility. Some (the bamboo shoots) will quickly learn to re-behave and reframe. Others will resist as if their very lives depended on it. When faced with an oak tree, the professional must do a good job of propping in hope that it will survive the hurricane.

Chapter 2

DESIGNING AND IMPLEMENTING A PROGRAM

This chapter is for those interested in developing a caregiver support program. If you have not yet established that your community needs a program of this kind, please refer to Neuber et al. (1980) for a discussion of need assessment techniques that may be helpful. Designing a program involves decisions ranging from the type of caregiver who will be eligible for the program to whether or not food will be served. This chapter presents suggestions based on the experiences reported by caregiver support efforts throughout the country. It presents specific issues to consider in advance, such as program objectives and target population, and concerns that arise during program implementation, such as recruiting caregivers, selecting a location, scheduling, transportation, respite care, and the dynamics of training sessions. Those interested in using the *Wellsprings* curriculum will find an overview of its sessions. The final section covers programming for special populations, such as rural caregivers, men caregivers, ethnic minorities, and isolated caregivers.

ESTABLISHING PROGRAM OBJECTIVES

Caregiver support programs can take many different forms and serve diverse objectives. I recommend the use of a broad or global goal, supported by more narrow, specific objectives. The goal of a program may be, for example, "to reduce caregiver distress" or "to prevent unnecessary nursing home utilization." A wide range of objectives might be used to reach these goals.

Objectives are most useful when they include an action and a measurable result. Here are some examples:

- to increase social support by teaching caregivers to communicate effectively with family, friends, and service providers
- to enhance caregivers' effectiveness by teaching them how to manage medications and adapt the home environment for patient safety
- to support the attainment of caregivers' personal goals through the use of individual coping plans

Regardless of the goal and objectives chosen, it is important that the outcome of the program be specific and measurable. This will help focus the intervention effort. The material presented in this book can be adapted to serve a wide range of objectives. The information and skills described in Chapters 5 through 9 should support behavioral change, stress management, and social support. The relaxation techniques presented in Appendix B directly support stress management, while the communication techniques presented there will enhance caregivers' ability to get the support they need. The self-care plan introduced in this chapter will enable caregivers to establish and work toward their goals. In addition to strengthening the intervention itself, specifying program outcomes will enhance evaluation efforts. Chapter 4 presents ways of measuring each of the goals and objectives listed above.

Determining the Target Population

It is important to give careful consideration to the target population that will be served by the program. Support groups for caregivers are often organized around a single disease, such as Alzheimer's or cancer. All members are coping with the same disease so information presented can focus on that common interest. This permits in-depth consideration of material that relates to the specific disease, but has several drawbacks. First, war stories from members dealing with the least common, most severe forms of a condition can frighten and depress participants who are dealing with a mild form. Further, those who have been recently diagnosed may become depressed when they encounter those dealing with an advanced condition. For example, a caregiver whose husband is in remission may find it difficult to hope for a cure when she is weekly confronted with someone whose remission has ended. Second, the overwhelming presence of a single disease as a source of commonality may lead caregivers to ignore more subtle, but equally important things that they have in common. For example, anyone providing care to a seriously ill loved one is likely to experience grief at the loss of the person they once knew. When sessions are organized around a single disease, there may not be time for discussion of this grief.

On the other hand, the diversity of a multi-disease group has both advantages and disadvantages. Disease-specific material is not appropriate for group meetings, so caregivers seeking this information must be referred elsewhere. But, exposure to a wide range of problem situations often reminds caregivers that theirs is not the worst possible form of human suffering without frightening them with the prospect that their situation might worsen.

A possible compromise between these two alternatives would be organizing groups that related to either a physical disability or a cognitive deficiency. So, those dealing with any form of dementia might be in one group, and those dealing with primarily physical problems might be in another. In some cases, the distinction may be hazy. For example, Parkinson's disease often combines physical disability with cognitive decline. Nonetheless, there is considerable evidence that additional stresses are associated with cognitive incapacity that may not necessarily come with physical disability (Eagles, Beattie, Blackwood, Restall, & Ashcroft, 1987; Zarit, Orr, & Zarit, 1985). The caregiver of a dementia victim typically confronts memory loss and behavioral problems that complicate the task of providing care. Separating caregivers of dementia victims from other caregivers can be justified on this basis.

A second decision regarding group formation is whether the relationship to the caregiver should be similar or different. That is, whether spouse caregivers should be separated from adult children and other caregivers. There is considerable evidence that husbands care differently from wives (Barusch & Spaid, 1989; Fitting & Rabins, 1985) and that adult children and spouses have different approaches to caregiving (Cantor, 1983; Toseland & Rossiter, 1989). In view of these differences it may be advisable to compose groups according to familial relationship (Toseland & Zarit, 1989). However, diversity in a group has some advantages. It sometimes enables group members to understand the feelings and behaviors of their family members. A spouse caregiver may gain insights from a daughter who can describe her reactions to the loss of a father.

Finally, those organizing a program for caregivers need to generate a precise definition of caregiving. One weakness of current work on caregiving is lack of consensus regarding the term's definition (Zarit & Toseland, 1989). Does caregiving mean hiring someone to take care of grandmother? Does it mean providing hands-on care around the clock? In the CSP program we required that participants provide at least 20 hours a day of direct care or supervision to the patient. This definition has the advantage of being easily communicated and measured. The 20-hour limit must be interpreted with some flexibility; however, so the person who provides only 19 and a half hours of care is not discouraged from participating. Until there is a broadly accepted definition of the term, programs must develop their own definitions in order to set eligibility guidelines.

RECRUITING CAREGIVERS

Recruiting efforts serve a dual purpose for programs of this type. They attract participants while introducing the project to the community at large. Due to isolation and independence, many caregivers present a challenge to recruiters. They tend to use few formal services and often view government help as welfare. For this reason, recruiting efforts require considerable time and effort.

These efforts will be enhanced if recruiting is considered while the program is being designed. As mentioned earlier, it is usually easier to recruit caregivers to participate in an educational program than to join a support group. As one CSP caregiver commented, "I just don't have time to sit around and listen to people complain." The title of the program, as well as material describing it might overcome this resistance by emphasizing the educational objectives. Once they are involved in the program caregivers will come to appreciate the value of peer support.

Early consideration should also be given to program auspices. Some public agencies carry a stigma that caregivers prefer to avoid. For example, many would be reluctant to participate in programs sponsored by the "Division for the Handicapped" or "Department of Mental Illness." Agencies with problematic titles may want to consider using the name of a subunit as the sponsoring entity or offering the program under the auspices of a different organization.

Recruiting caregivers requires persistent and diverse efforts. Generally, it is unwise to rely on a single source for all referrals. In part, this is because few sources will provide the number of caregivers necessary to sustain an independent program. In addition, reliance on a single source will reduce the diversity of caregivers served. CSP relied on agency referral, media, word of mouth, and neighborhood canvassing. Table 2.1 shows the percentage of CSP participants recruited from each source.

Working with Agencies

Such agencies as senior centers, home health agencies, senior day care facilities, nursing and rehabilitation centers, and Area Agencies on Aging are particularly helpful in referring appropriate group members. Presentations about the support group to agencies' staffs can be an effective way to heighten awareness of the program. Another alternative is delivering an in-service training session on a topic related to caregiving or stress management. By providing training, recruiters can both establish themselves as experts and develop reciprocal relationships with agency staff. Alternatively, staff from key programs can be invited to address the caregivers during a relevant session.

The key to effective agency referral is establishing strong, personal relationships with agency staff. The staff needs constant reminders that the program is available. They also need feedback on what happened with the people they referred. The use of weekly phone calls and identification of an agency mediator who will remind staff at meetings or on a casual basis will be helpful. It also may be helpful to establish an advisory board made up of staff members from key agencies.

Some service providers need to get formal written consent from caregivers to make a referral. This is necessary to protect their clients' privacy. It is important to make this process as easy as possible for the provider in order to facilitate referrals. Some agencies already have the necessary release forms. Others might prefer to mail your recruiting material themselves. One option to consider is encouraging a staff member or caregiver to do volunteer work in a key agency. In this capacity, the volunteer will have access to clients and, with agency approval, may inform clients about the caregiver program.

Table 2.1
Source of CSP Referrals

	Percentages	
Agencies		
Hospital-based home care, V.A.	16	
Area Agency on Aging	13	
Community home health services	7	
Senior citizen centers	7	
Churches	3	
Gerontology list	3	
Other agencies	3	
Subtotal		52
Media		
Newspapers	18	
Television	2	
Radio	1	
Poster/Pamphlet	1	
Other	1	
Subtotal		23
Word Of Mouth		
Staff	10	
Project caregivers	11	
Family	3	
Other	2	
Subtotal		26

Using the Media

The public media are the best means of achieving public awareness, as most people have access to newspaper, radio, and television. Also, a certain amount of credibility is associated with the media. Feature articles and press releases submitted to newspapers and local newsletters are excellent ways to notify the public of the program. For CSP, newspapers were the single most effective recruiting approach, yielding 18% of participants. Public service announcements, television and radio talk shows, and interviews are good avenues to gain referrals.

Posters and Pamphlets

Posters and pamphlets also can be used to publicize a program. CSP distributed posters and pamphlets through mass mailings and displays. Mailings to churches proved fruitful, and several pharmacies and clinics displayed pamphlets at central locations. Pharmacists were especially helpful, encouraging their patients to pick up pamphlets and use the training. Physicians were less likely to encourage participation. Posters were displayed in a variety of locations: hospitals, clinics, pharmacies, and senior high-rise complexes. Posters were most effective when used in conjunction with pamphlets.

The pamphlets remain as concrete reminders of the program and offer interested persons all the relevant facts in a concise manner. One CSP caregiver picked up a pamphlet in her doctor's office, put it up on her refrigerator, and thought about calling for 3 months. She finally got up the courage to call and became involved in the program.

Word of Mouth

Word of mouth can eventually serve as an excellent source of referrals, so recruiting efforts should not be targeted only toward the elderly. Often family members of caregivers will see information about the project and then pass it on to the parent, sibling, or adult child. Participants who have completed the program also may be able to pass on names of potential group members.

Neighborhood Canvassing

Door-to-door canvassing in neighborhoods with high-density elderly populations is another option. While it may raise awareness, this approach is not recommended. Most elderly are suspicious of strangers who knock on their doors, expecting them to be salespeople or solicitors at best. CSP staff found canvassing time-consuming, threatening, and inefficient.

Although a wide-ranging recruiting effort does require time and effort, it will increase the pool of available participants. Diverse recruiting efforts sometimes have a cumulative effect. Someone who was referred through an Area Agency on Aging might ultimately agree to participate because he or she had already heard about the project on a radio interview.

Once a caregiver is aware that training is available, various issues may keep him or her from getting involved in a group. These issues need to be addressed by the coordinators. They include location, scheduling, transportation, and respite care.

SELECTING A LOCATION

It is best to hold the group meetings in a central location in the community. A central location is within more caregivers' reach and is easier to find. CSP, for example, did not hold any groups at the University of Utah. The university is not centrally located, nor is it familiar to the elderly. Excellent locations include public libraries, senior centers, nursing homes and home health agencies, community extension centers, senior high-rise complexes, adult mobile home parks, club houses, and church meeting rooms. Because any location will be undesirable for some caregivers organizers planning to hold several training groups may prefer to vary their location. So, for example, one group might meet in a library and the next in a senior center. Those who indicate they cannot attend in one location can then be referred to a group meeting somewhere else.

Public libraries provide easy access and a quiet setting. The librarian may be willing to put up a display of caregiver help books. Some libraries have regulations that require all meetings to be open to the public. You may or may not be willing to take the chance of having someone drop in on your group.

Senior centers offer a positive environment for the group. Members may get an enlightened view of the advantages of being involved in a center and negative stereotypes may be broken down.

Nursing homes and home health agencies are usually happy to cooperate in providing an available meeting room. This exposes their business to the population most likely to need it. For caregivers, meeting in a nursing home can help reduce their anxiety about using a long-term care facility. However, those who have never been in a nursing home may have some fears that might prevent them from attending.

Table 2.2 presents some considerations to keep in mind when selecting a meeting place.

Table 2.2

Considerations in Selecting a Meeting Place

---

(1) Find a quiet area for the least possible distractions.

(2) Choose a room that is wheelchair accessible and, if necessary, has a working elevator.

(3) The building and room should be easy to locate. You may want to put out signs with arrows for the first few sessions. Provide clear written directions to participants, showing where they will park.

(4) Make sure there is ample parking.

(5) Inform the receptionist at each group location about the group times and room number so he or she can help direct participants.

(6) Be sure the room is the appropriate size for the number in your group. Too large or too small a room can be uncomfortable.

(7) Be sure there are chairs in the room and that they are set up. Consider arranging the chairs in a circle to encourage interaction.

(8) Be wary of an overcrowded room with lots of tables and chairs. (Tables tend to reduce intimacy, and empty chairs look abandoned.)

(9) If the building has a public address system with regular announcements, see whether it can be turned off in the group meeting room.

(10) Do preparations when using slides and films. Ensure that the projector and screen are available and that the lighting can be dimmed.

(11) Finding a place can be a challenge. Rooms may not be available. Food may not be allowed. Ask other people who are running community groups for recommendations.

SCHEDULING

The time a group is held will influence participation. Many caregivers do not like to drive after 5:00 p.m. due to rush hour traffic, night blindness, and care receivers' needs for extra attention in the evening. Staff of most agencies that provide respite for caregivers do not work in the evening. In contrast, those caregivers who rely on family for transportation and respite prefer to wait until evening. Morning is generally a difficult time to meet. There are several advantages to meeting in the afternoon. In the winter, snow and ice are often removed or melted by 1:00 p.m. Respite support is usually more available in the afternoon. Many care receivers need less care in the afternoon and can be left alone then.

TRANSPORTATION

Providing transportation will enhance participation. Some caregivers cannot or will not drive during certain times of the day, as mentioned above. Caregivers should be encouraged to use their support systems and accept offers from friends and neighbors for both transportation and respite. Learning to accept help is a milestone for most caregivers. Alternatively, many use their support systems extensively and are reluctant to ask for more help, particularly when it involves doing something for themselves. Caregivers who drive may be willing to provide transportation for other participants. Area Agencies on Aging may be aware of volunteer drivers or senior transportation that could be used. The local bus service may be convenient for the caregiver. Group leaders may be able to pick up group members, but this should be viewed as a last resort. Usually group leaders need to arrive early to set up and to stay late to talk individually with members.

RESPITE CARE

A caregiver may need someone to stay with the care receiver while he or she attends group meetings. Family members may be working or caring for their children, or they may not live close enough to provide respite. Caregivers should participate in efforts to identify possible respite providers. Initially it is usually best to consider informal sources of help, such as family and friends. Church staff may coordinate weekly volunteers. Sometimes a motivated, caring neighbor will agree to organize neighborhood volunteers.

When informal sources of respite are unavailable, consider using local service providers. Locally sponsored respite programs, such as the Senior Companion program, may offer a companion for those who are homebound. Adult day-care centers may be a good option. Respite often provides a positive experience for the care receiver by offering a chance to interact with and trust another person. This begins the process of resource utilization and allows the caregiver to have time away and begin to trust that others can be responsible for giving care. In some cases, an electronic device, such as Life Line, may be hooked up so the homebound family member can contact a neighbor in case of an emergency.

RELUCTANT CAREGIVERS

Many caregivers are reluctant to participate in support programs. The recruiter's task in working with a reluctant caregiver is to identify and attempt to resolve any problems that inhibit participation. Reluctance should be addressed directly and with respect. The caregiver probably has good reasons to hesitate. The recruiter who responds to those reasons positively, saying, in essence, "I can see why you would hesitate to participate. Let's see if we can make it easier for you to do so," will increase the likelihood that the caregiver will participate in and benefit from the program.

Causes of reluctance vary: Some caregivers may not understand the nature of the program and its potential benefits; other caregivers may not want to "make a bad situation worse" by risking any change; still others may feel too overwhelmed to take on yet another commitment; and care receivers may resist the program, for a variety of reasons.

Both caregiver and care receiver may have mistaken ideas about the nature of a caregiver support program. If the recruiter suspects this may be the case a personal visit from a group leader might be helpful. Explaining the purpose and benefits of the group will help both people to feel better about their involvement. Caregivers can be encouraged to share what they learn from the group with their ill family member. The caregiver might be willing to attend the first session on a trial basis. This would enable him or her to make an informed decision about participating. If the caregiver agrees to a trial visit, the recruiter should schedule a follow-up discussion. This might include both the caregiver and the care receiver. If the caregiver chooses not to continue with the program it is important to learn his or her reasons. They may indicate problems with the program that can be solved in later sessions, or individual concerns that can be addressed.

Caregivers who hesitate to "make a bad situation worse" are expressing a natural ambivalence. We are all ambivalent about change.

We want to grow and improve, but we also cling to the status quo as the best known alternative. The program will involve a significant investment of time and effort and there are no guarantees that it will help. It might even make things worse. The recruiter may recognize and acknowledge this ambivalence, helping the caregiver to weigh the costs of participating against the potential benefits. A tentative decision to participate might be the caregiver's first step toward overcoming this ambivalence.

The overwhelmed caregiver is most likely to need the support offered by a program and may be most reluctant to participate. When all of a person's energy is consumed with caring for a loved one it is virtually impossible to contemplate making a commitment to a caregiver program. Caregivers who are overwhelmed often feel that they are indispensable. They are trying to do everything for their loved one and jeopardizing their health and well-being in the process. In this situation caregivers worry about what would happen if they became ill or died before the care receiver did. This worry might motivate them to participate in a support program. A successful recruiting effort might address this concern, pointing out that the program will help caregivers identify other resources to support their loved one, even as it enhances their well-being.

A care receiver may resist the program for several reasons. He or she may be emotionally dependent on the caregiver and resist separation. The care receiver may fear that the program will encourage the caregiver to place him or her in a nursing home. The care receiver who feels especially vulnerable may try to control the caregiver's activities and decisions. Because outside allegiances might reduce this control, the prospect of a support program can be threatening to a care receiver in this situation. In dealing with the care receiver's concerns the same general rule applies: They should be addressed directly and with respect. Ultimately the decision to participate rests with the caregiver. By addressing the care receiver's concerns the recruiter will go far toward ensuring the caregiver's successful participation.

Unfortunately the recruiter will sometimes have to just accept a caregiver's refusal to participate. If this is done in good grace it can set the stage for future participation if circumstances (or opinions) change. In some situations, individual training may be advisable. CSP has pioneered an individual approach to caregiver training, which is described later in this chapter.

TRAINING DYNAMICS

Caregivers are usually emotionally healthy persons who can use extra skills and information to manage their situation. A support program is an excellent context for meeting these needs. Nonetheless, programs like *Wellsprings* that focus on skills training do have limitations. As Lazarus and Folkman (1984) pointed out, skills training can fail "because of longstanding personal difficulties involving conflicts, hidden agendas, and fears originating early in life that have been continually reinforced and maintained by later patterns of living, or from pervasive beliefs in one's inadequacy" (p. 368). Clearly a short-term training program is not the appropriate context for addressing problems of this kind. Individuals who want help with such issues may do best when referred for individual counseling or ongoing group therapy.

Selecting a Group Leader

Selecting a group leader is an important consideration. Groups can be led by either lay leaders or professionals. In their 1989 study, Toseland and colleagues reported that each approach proved effective (Toseland, Rossiter, & Labrecque, 1989a). Lay leaders were more likely to encourage socializing, sharing personal experiences, and ventilating feelings. Professional leaders tended to be somewhat more effective at keeping discussions focused on caregiving issues. They tended to introduce greater structure and use a more active leadership style.

The best approach might be to have two leaders: one a lay person with experience in caregiving, the other a professional. When one leader is presenting material or leading discussion, the other can attend to the group's response. The nonpresenter can request clarification when the group seems lost, or identify individuals who are having trouble with the material. A male and female combination is helpful as some people may relate best to one or the other sex. In addition, leaders should use different yet complementary styles of communication. At first, co-leaders will find it helpful to practice one session on other staff and then discuss the quality of their interaction and presentation.

Managing the Group

Even in an educational forum, group-work skills can be helpful. Group leaders need to maintain control of the group process. Some members may have needs that cannot be met within the group context. Some may monopolize the conversation. In these situations, it is important to be assertive and possibly to confront the group member involved. The leader must direct the conversation back to the subject. The leader may need to say, for example, "I can see how this is difficult for you. We really need to continue with the session, then we can talk about this after group." Group leaders cannot allow one person to jeopardize the positive group experience for everyone else.

Leaders also should monitor their personal reactions to group members. Some members may "get under the skin" of the leader. In this case, leaders should work together. Each co-leader might take responsibility for working with the individual during a specific session. The group's need to maintain focus must be balanced against the value of spontaneous discussion of important or timely topics. Although leaders must be prepared with a clear agenda, they must be equally prepared to abandon that agenda. Group members' own agenda should sometimes take precedence.

A combination of teaching and supportive interaction is very effective in caregiver support programs. Group interaction provides an opportunity to illustrate the use of various communication techniques and to clarify training concepts. Often, personal growth will come from recognizing a feeling or problem described by someone else. The group interaction serves to validate and legitimize feelings, as a caregiver realizes that he or she is not the only person who feels a certain way. Group leaders should seek to facilitate emotional support between group members. This can be done by encouraging participants to exchange telephone numbers and socialize outside of the group. Exercises that use dyads or small groups can also encourage supportive relationships within the group.

Training presentations should access several senses: auditory, visual, and sensory. This will enhance understanding of the issues being explored. The auditory sense might be accessed through a lecture or discussion. Visual material might be presented using film, slides, or overheads. Sensory experiences, such as writing notes or filling in blanks, will also support learning. Experiential activities are also effective. These include exercises, such as wearing cotton in the ears or smearing glasses with vaseline, that are designed to promote empathy for those with sensory impairments. Other exercises give caregivers a chance to practice new communication and relaxation skills in small groups.

Using a Self-Care Plan

Many training programs are designed to enhance caregivers' coping abilities. A self-care plan can be used to accomplish this goal. The plan can be introduced by acknowledging how often caregivers feel powerless. Caregivers can be encouraged to provide individual examples of how they feel when they feel powerless. The self-care plan is introduced as a way of taking just a little bit of control of the situation.

The self-care plan presented here is adapted from the action plan presented in "Growing Wiser" published by Healthwise Incorporated. This plan gives each caregiver an opportunity to be selfish. Leaders should emphasize the "healthiness of selfishness" and make it a rule that caregivers be entirely selfish in designing and carrying out the self-care plan. The plan's goals must directly benefit not the patient but the caregiver. It may be helpful to remind caregivers that by meeting their own needs they will enhance their ability to provide care to their loved ones. With this brief introduction of the plan, the leader will describe the steps involved in developing and carrying out a self-care plan. There are six steps involved.

SELF-CARE PLAN: SIX STEPS

Step 1: Identify a problem. Participants will be encouraged to identify personal problems that relate to their caregiving situation. The leader should identify a personal problem that he or she would like to work on, such as not having enough free time, and use that to illustrate the following steps. Caregivers in CSP identified problems such as lack of privacy, fatigue, lack of fun, and anxiety.

Step 2: Specify a goal. Again, the goal must be selfish—it must be for the benefit of the caregiver. In this example, the leader's goal might be to set aside some personal time. The goal should be stated in positive, as opposed to negative, terms. That is, it should be to achieve a desired state, not to eliminate an undesired one. This provides an opportunity to demonstrate reframing as a technique. For example, the lack of free time might yield a negative goal to stop feeling so overwhelmed and rushed, or it might yield a positive goal to feel more relaxed and in charge. By focusing on the positive goal, the caregiver is directing all of his or her energy toward a desired future. By its reference to an unpleasant past, a negative goal can undermine successful progress.

Step 3: Describe a specific outcome. The caregiver will indicate a specific objective, which is measurable. In this example, an objective might be to save Monday morning for free time.

Step 4: Identify action steps and barriers. These action steps should be small and doable. In our example, they might include turning off the phone Monday mornings or blocking out Monday morning on a calendar. Once the action steps are identified, participants list barriers that might prevent them from succeeding. One might, for example, feel guilty about turning off the phone or find it impossible to save time on a calendar. Problem solving can be used at this point to discuss means of overcoming these barriers. Friends and environmental changes might be used to overcome the barriers. In this example, a friend might call just to see whether the leader has taken her free time this week.

Step 5: Visualization. Visualization is an important part of a self-care plan. Research has consistently shown the effectiveness of visualization for changing behavior. People who see themselves engaged in an activity are not only more likely to engage in that activity later, they are also likely to do better when they do. So caregivers are encouraged to visualize themselves succeeding in action steps. Our leader might imagine calmly lounging next to the coffee table Monday morning. Visualization also can help identify barriers and initiate the problem-solving process described earlier.

Step 6: Reporting. Caregivers report each week on their progress in reaching self-care goals. The reporting time is not an opportunity for self-criticism. Instead, it provides caregivers with some support and help with problem solving to enhance the next week's efforts. CSP has developed a form for monitoring self-care plans. This is presented at the end of this chapter.

Guest Speakers

Guest speakers can be a valuable part of a group session. A guest can address an issue related to a specific area of expertise. This also gives caregivers an opportunity to meet someone in the community who may later serve as a resource. The group leaders need to screen guest speakers and prepare them for the group's style. Guests should not request that each member introduce him- or herself and describe the caregiving situation. This is redundant for the members and seldom necessary for the guest. Guests should not take up the entire group time, because their presentation may not be significant to every member. A guest speaker may not have the skills to facilitate a group. If discussion gets intense or heated, group leaders need to be involved to keep the situation appropriate.

Dysfunctional Participants

Leaders should always be aware of any caregiver who seems highly dysfunctional and check for signs of pathological or potentially abusive situations. In these situations, leaders should consider referring the member to available support for his or her specific need. (See Quinn & Tomita, 1986, for a detailed discussion of assessment and intervention in situations involving elder abuse or neglect.)

Details

Many details contribute to a quality experience. For both leaders and members, beginning and ending on time creates an expectation of promptness and shows respect for those who are prompt. It also helps to ensure enough time to cover each session's agenda. Each member should be urged to attend the first session. Initial introductions begin a crucial rapport within the group. In addition, group rules are clarified and the tone is set. It is difficult for a member to join in if he or she missed the initial session, so leaders may want to refer that member to a later group.

Name tags are a valuable tool. They personalize interaction immediately between leaders and members. Tags also reduce the stress of trying to recall someone's name.

If equipment is to be used, leaders must check on its availability in advance. Some group locations may have equipment that they will allow the group to use. Leaders must be sure the equipment, including electrical outlets and extension cords, is working.

It is always beneficial for the leaders to listen to and process constructive feedback from members so that they can continually improve the group. When a group runs smoothly and leaders have adequately prepared, all involved will have a positive experience.

The *Wellsprings* Curriculum

Table 2.3 provides an outline of the seven-session *Wellsprings* training program. The sessions combine didactic presentation with related exercises. Each one takes 2 hours, with a 15-minute break and related exercises. Relaxation and communication exercises are presented in Appendix B. Each session should close with a relaxation exercise. Communication skills can be practiced in dyads, then couples can report to the entire group. All sessions include homework assignments. It is important that participants report on their homework and self-care plans at the beginning of each session.

Closure

If the program is time limited, it is important to prepare both leaders and participants for closure. Trainers may want to make a continuing support group available, either by referring participants to an existing group or by establishing a new group. Of course, not all caregivers need or want a support group. A member may not want a continued group, but may ask to be referred to a counselor. Or, a caregiver may just want to know that resources are available in the future for questions or dilemmas.

The main purpose of short-term training is not to provide support but to enable caregivers to find and create support for themselves. Through training, caregivers feel more assertive and confident in meeting their needs. They learn how to use the system to make their situation better.

PROGRAMMING FOR SPECIAL POPULATIONS

Rural Caregivers

America's elderly are concentrated in small towns in rural areas of this country. These areas have the highest proportion of elderly (15.4% of the local population), compared to urban and suburban areas, which have about 10% (Krout, 1986). Frail elderly in rural areas face a well-documented shortage of medical and social services (Nelson, 1980; Palmore, 1983). Yet they choose to remain in familiar surroundings, with the support of family and friends.

Table 2.3

Overview of *Wellsprings* Sessions

Session	Content	Leader Concerns

1	Introductions
	Self-Care Plans
		Support individual
		  contributions—prevent one
		  participant from monopolizing
		  the session

	Relaxation: Deep breathing	Set tone for future sessions
	Communication: Assertiveness	End on up-beat note
	HOMEWORK: Self-care, deep breathing	

2	Report on self-care plans
	Normal aging
	Relaxation: Muscle
	  relaxation
	Communication: Fogging
		Prevent self-criticism by
		  those who do not progress
		Emphasize relevance of material

	HOMEWORK: Self-care and fogging	

3	Report on self-care plans
	Emotional Needs
	Communication:
	  Negative assertion and
	  negative inquiry
	Relaxation: Crisis breathing
		Encourage recognition of unmet
		  needs of both caregiver and
		  care receiver

	HOMEWORK: Self-care and crisis breathing	

4	Report on self-care plans
	Community resources
	Communication: Broken
	  record
	Relaxation: Chinese breath
		Select and prepare guest speaker
		  (staff of public agency)
		Direct participants' frustration
		  with service inadequacies toward
		  policymakers and service provider

	HOMEWORK: Self-care, contact one service provider	

5	Report on self-care plans
	Legal & financial concerns
	Communication: Workable
	  compromise
	Relaxation: Instant
	  relaxation (3,2,1)
		Select and prepare guest speaker
		Remind caregivers to bring
		  medications for session 6
		Minimize sense of helplessness
		  when faced with legal
		  technicalities

	HOMEWORK: Self-care and workable compromise	

(continued)

Rural communities pose several challenges for efforts in support of caregivers. Great distances make group meetings problematic, and the

Table 2.3 (continued)

Session	Content	Leader Concerns

6	Report on self-care plans
	Caregiving skills
	Communication: DESC
	  scripting
	Relaxation: Visualization
		Select and prepare guest speaker
		  (pharmacist)
		Support caregivers' sense of
		  efficacy

	HOMEWORK:	Self-care and visualization

7	Report on self-care plans
	Grief and mourning
	Exercise: Letting go
	Relaxation: Massage
		Closure—encourage planning for
		  self-care, identify continuing
		  support groups, support
		  networking
		Permission for grieving

	HOMEWORK:	Deciding to live

absence of service providers can complicate transportation and respite arrangements. Yet several organizations have managed to develop successful caregiver support programs by making optimal use of the resources available in rural areas. Successful programs seem to have two things in common: They involve local leadership, and they stress social support and personal contact (Beisecker, 1989).

Two programs illustrate the range of approaches to serving rural caregivers. The Volunteer Information Provider Program (VIPP) is a nationwide effort that uses the Cooperative Extension Service to train volunteers who then provide information to caregivers. Local volunteers receive training in a variety of topics through the extension service. They then provide information and emotional support to caregivers in their communities. The VIPP program uses no audiovisual material or expert presenters in recognition of the scarcity of resources in rural areas. In contrast, the Western Kentucky University Caregiver Project provides information to caregivers using videotapes and teleconferencing. In this project, a network of local volunteers organize simultaneous meetings of caregivers, where videotapes were shown. Following each tape, teleconferencing enables caregivers to interact with a member of the university faculty.

The VIPP program proves the effectiveness of working with the county extension service. The extension service has a long history of providing educational services in rural areas. Within the service, the county home economist may be most interested in working on care-giver programs. This nationwide network can be a great resource for caregiver support. Extension offices are usually listed under "County Offices" in local telephone directories.

Programming for rural areas should make use of the unique strengths of these areas while taking into account their unique dif-ficulties. One strength is the strong informal support system found in most rural areas. As a result, nontraditional referral sources, such as the mail carrier, can serve as gatekeepers, helping to inform care-givers of programs. In order to make the best use of these strong in-formal systems local leaders should participate in planning and, if possible, implementing the program. On the other hand, the distances that separate residents in rural areas can preclude face-to-face meetings. The telephone might be used to overcome this difficulty, with a network of caregivers sharing support and information. The lack of formal services poses another difficulty in most rural areas. Programs will not have extensive resources for transportation and respite available. Often, strong informal supports will compensate for the lack of formal services, as neighbors, family, and friends help meet transportation and respite needs.

Men Caregivers

In many ways, the needs and concerns of male caregivers are just the same as those of women who provide care. At the risk of en-couraging stereotypes, we can identify some concerns shared by many male caregivers. Usually men are more reluctant than women to participate in support groups. Drs. Kaye and Applegate recently com-pleted a study of male caregivers, reported in a book entitled *Men as Care-givers to the Elderly* (Kaye and Applegate, 1990). He and his colleagues have identified some barriers that deter men from becom-ing involved in caregiver support groups. One barrier is an inconveni-ent meeting time. Male caregivers are more likely to be employed, so daytime meetings may be impossible for them to attend. Inappropriate sponsorship may be another barrier. Men may be reluctant, for example, to participate in a group that is sponsored by the YWCA. Subtle factors might encourage men to participate. For example, men could be mentioned in any PSAs or advertisements about the program. If in-dividual contacts are used for recruiting, men could contact other men. Having a man serve as leader or co-leader for a group might enhance male participation. Kaye and his colleagues also suggest that men may prefer a program that offers practical information to one that focuses on emotional support. Emphasis on expert speakers and useful information might draw men into the group so that they can enjoy the emotional benefits of participation. Finally, the individual format described below may appeal to men who are unwilling to join a group.

Isolated Caregivers

Many caregivers are unwilling or unable to leave their loved ones to attend a group meeting. CSP experienced initial problems recruiting caregivers for training groups. In analyzing caregivers' reasons for refusal, we found that many were simply unwilling or unable to leave their spouses. These caregivers did not feel comfortable leaving their spouses for a few hours even if they had respite and transportation available. Others lacked resources for respite or transportation. These homebound caregivers are especially vulnerable to stress given their total commitment to caring and their isolation. To respond to the needs of this group, an individual training program was developed to provide training in caregivers' homes.

The content of the training sessions was the same as that of the group sessions, but the process was quite different. Group sessions allowed several members to discuss their experiences and problems. In the home setting, each caregiver had greater opportunity to speak about his or her situation. Although some enjoyed this exclusive interaction, they did miss the camaraderie offered by a group.

The individual format presents several challenges. It is occasionally difficult to keep the professional distance that allows for objective teaching and exploration of the caregiving situation. Meeting in the privacy of someone's home offers a more personal atmosphere for training. This informality may tempt both caregivers and trainers to focus on particular problems and not on the training agenda. It is important that the in-home trainer both listen to the caregiver and guide the conversation back to the training agenda. For example, when a caregiver begins to complain about an adult child who criticizes, the trainer might take the opportunity to demonstrate a learned conversation skill that deals with criticism.

Many caregivers will begin to see the trainer as a friend and anticipate a continuing relationship after training ends. This may prove difficult for the trainer who needs to bring closure. The point of the training is to enhance the caregiver's independence and self-care. Rathe than providing a needed relationship, the trainer will offer each caregive the skills needed to initiate such relationships elsewhere.

In the home setting, interruptions are inevitable. The ill spous may need attention, the phone may ring, and someone who has nc come to visit for a long time may drop by. Advance discussion of hov interruptions will be handled will ease this situation. Caregiver an trainer may set limits on their willingness to tolerate interruptior Phones do not have to be answered, nor do doorbells. Still, it is some times appropriate to end training for the day and come back later t finish the session or to continue the session at the next appointment.

Individual sessions provide training and support to caregivers wh would otherwise be unable to receive services—those who are so er meshed in caregiving or so overwhelmed with duties that they cannc even break away to attend a group. Another advantage of the individua option is that the trainer can personalize the material to the caregiver' situation. More time can be taken to process information. Often, care givers feel more free to ask questions in a one-to-one setting.

The individual format can be expensive. Few programs have th luxury of assigning a trained social worker to provide training to in dividual caregivers. With volunteers, the cost-effectiveness of in dividual training might be increased. Professional staff might trai and supervise older volunteers (perhaps former caregivers) who the provide training and support. This model proved effective for the VIP described above. It holds promise for serving isolated caregivers.

Ethnic Minorities

Ethnic minorities are underrepresented among participants of care giver support groups (Toseland & Zarit, 1989); most participants i these groups are white and middle-class. Targeted recruiting effort might draw minority caregivers into support groups. Unless th groups have been tailored to serve minorities, these caregivers ar likely to be alienated. This is because the family dynamics that forn the backdrop for caregiving are largely the products of cultura traditions and expectations. Even the most sensitive group facilitato will occasionally misunderstand the nuances of a situation that i foreign to his or her cultural background.

This is not to discourage programmers from recruiting minorit caregivers, but to suggest that we go beyond recruiting to deliberate programming to meet the needs of this population. Programming in support of minority caregivers will first employ minority staff as group leaders, trainers and counselors. Once this step, the most important one, has been taken, caregiver programs can be restructured to various degrees in response to local needs. Options to consider include relocating group meetings to be closer to ethnic communities, conducting part or all of the meeting in the native language of the minority group, providing bilingual written material, assigning companions to minority caregivers to help with translation and participation (such as other minority caregivers who are assimilated into the dominant culture), inviting guest speakers who are leaders in the minority community (religious leaders, as well as professional leaders), and holding subgroup meetings for minority caregivers.

RESOURCES

Determining the Need for a Caregiver Support Program:

Neuber, K.A., & Associates (1980). *Needs assessment: A model for community planning.* Beverly Hills, CA: Sage.

Programming for Rural Populations:

The Center on Rural Elderly's Compendium of Educational Materials includes a review of caregiver programs. It is available by contacting:

Center on Rural Elderly
University of Missouri—Kansas City
5245 Rockhill Road
Kansas City, MO 64110
(816) 276-2180

For more information on the VIPP:

Bane, S., & Halpert, B.P. (1986). *Instructor's manual information for caregivers of the elderly.* Kansas City: Center for Aging Studies, University of Missouri—Kansas City.

Bane, S., & Halpert, B.P. (1986). *Resource manual information for caregivers of the elderly.* Kansas City: Center on Aging Studies, University of Missouri—Kansas City.

Chapter 3

EVALUATING PROGRAM EFFECTIVENESS

Anyone who operates a caregiver program should devote some effort to evaluation. The practice of caregiver support is in its infancy. Several programs have been developed and evaluated with various degrees of rigor. But we still know very little about what works for caregivers and why. Through systematic evaluation a program can contribute to our understanding of this growing field. Evaluation efforts also can improve the program itself. Finally, data on effectiveness can be used to secure funding for a program's continuation or expansion.

Resistance to evaluation takes many forms. For some, the word evaluation conjures up images of multi-million dollar designs, sophisticated statistics, and elaborate computer software, all to demonstrate that the program had no discernable effect. This chapter is based on my belief that worthwhile evaluation efforts can be operated on a shoestring budget and without a computer! Further, I will argue that there is no such thing as a negative evaluation.

Evaluation can be used to assess both the process and the outcome of a program. Process evaluation answers the following questions: What did we really do? To whom? How often? Outcome evaluation answers the question, Did the program meet its goals and objectives? When both process and outcome evaluation are conducted another set of questions can be addressed: What aspect of the program was particularly useful? Who was most likely to benefit from this program?

EVALUATING THE PROCESS

If programs operated according to plan there would be no need for process evaluation. We could answer the process question, "What did we do?" simply by referring to the program brochure or outline. Having spent hundreds of hours designing a caregiver program it may be inconceivable that the program would not operate according to plan. But, as any veteran in the human services knows, it will not. Clients will be admitted who do not meet all eligibility criteria. Clients will participate in some but not all of the training sessions. They will sleep through a session or, worse, they will drop out after the third session. Workers will quit. Some sessions just will not go according to the agenda. We need process evaluation simply to keep track of the minor and major deviations from the plan (or, in an ideal case, to document our strict adherence to the plan).

Process evaluation involves routinely monitoring key program elements. These may include:

- Referral source: How do most clients learn about the program?
- Client characteristics: Age, gender, relation to the care receiver, employment status, health status, motivation for caregiving
- Client participation: Attendance and degree of involvement—for those who drop out, Why?
- Worker characteristics: Age, gender, caregiving experience, educational background
- Service characteristics: Dynamics of each session or interaction—Do some people call between sessions to problem-solve with staff? Do some sessions seem to bomb, while others generate enthusiastic participation?

There is a tendency, particularly among those operating small programs to expect to remember everything that happened. While memory does serve well in some areas, our recall of an event can be colored by subsequent events. When Mrs. X drops out of training we tend to remember that she never seemed interested in the material presented. Referring to process documents may remind us that she was passionately interested but always seemed very tired when she arrived for a session.

The CSP program used screening forms and session notes for process evaluation. These forms are included at the end of this chapter (see Tables 3.1 and 3.3). We were interested in clients who dropped out after attending only a few sessions. After each training program we called the dropouts (if there were any) and asked why they had stopped participating. We also asked whether there was anything about the program that could be changed to better suit their needs. When staff are not available to make these phone calls a caregiver who has successfully completed the training program might do so. The information they yield may be reassuring. Caregivers in the CSP program tended to report that they dropped out because of a change in their life circumstances, not dissatisfaction with the program. Of course, most caregivers are reluctant to criticize a program. (This is one reason why it is best if group leaders do not make the phone calls.) Information collected should be interpreted with that in mind.

EVALUATING THE OUTCOME

Outcome evaluations measure the extent to which the program met its goals and objectives. They dare human service professionals to prove their worth. Because of this, outcome evaluations can be intimidating. Yet, if done properly, these evaluations cannot produce negative results. Even if the answer to the question "Did it really work?" is a resounding "No!" knowledge of how to (and how not to) intervene in support of caregivers will be gained. Results of outcome evaluations are seldom as concrete as that. More likely will be the finding that intervention works sometimes, or just a little, or for some people and not for others. These ambiguous answers, while not as satisfying as a robust "Yes," can be useful.

The primary goal in selecting an *evaluation design* is to minimize the extent to which the findings will be ambiguous or contaminated. That is, if results suggest that participants improved, the design should minimize the number of alternative explanations for the improvement. This will enable the evaluator to attribute the change to the program rather than to other extraneous factors. There are three main approaches to outcome evaluation: *experimental designs, quasi-experimental designs,* and *client satisfaction surveys.* Experimental designs are characterized by the use of a true control group. These designs are the most likely to produce uncontaminated results. Quasi-experimental designs employ comparison groups, and typically fail to eliminate some alternate explanations of findings. Client satisfaction surveys, often called "smile-o-meters," are the least objective approach to outcome evaluation. They are discussed here because the results they produce are often valuable to program advocates.

EXPERIMENTAL DESIGNS

A true *experimental design* is one in which individuals are randomly assigned to treatment and control groups. *Random assignment* exists when each participant has an equal chance of being assigned to any group. If you have a list of participants to begin with, this might be done with a random number table. Each person on the list can be assigned a number, and the numbers are then divided evenly between groups according to a pre-established rule. For example, even numbers go into the control group and odd numbers into a training program.

Sometimes programs do not have a list of eligible participants. Instead, caregivers may trickle into the program, with one or two calling each day in response to recruiting efforts. Then they can be individually assigned by tossing a coin, rolling a die or dice, or using any similar random procedure. For example, caregivers might be randomly assigned to either a control group or a training group by using a coin toss. When a caregiver calls to ask about the training program staff would first determine eligibility, then toss a coin. "heads" would mean assignment to the control group, and "tails" would send him or her to a training group. The same procedure could be used to assign people to different training groups if you were interested in comparing their effectiveness.

Matching procedures can be used when the evaluator suspects that some key factor or factors may influence a client's outcome. If, for example, research has indicated (as it has) that men experience considerably less burden as caregivers than do women, you might view gender as one of these key factors. To ensure an equal number of men and women in the groups you would assign each man or woman a partner. Then toss a coin to decide which of the pair would go into which group. Thus the groups would be matched for gender.

Professionals committed to serving caregivers often find the procedures associated with random assignment offensive. It is extremely difficult to tell a caregiver who is under enormous stress that he or she has been assigned to a control group. It is also difficult to secure referrals from community agencies when there is a 50% likelihood that the client referred will not receive services. Further, caregivers who are assigned to a control group are likely to drop out of the program altogether, refusing contact with program staff. For these and related reasons, quasi-experimental designs are often used to assess the outcome of caregiver programs.

QUASI-EXPERIMENTAL DESIGNS

Unlike experimental designs, which enable us to control for possible intervening forces, quasi-experimental designs simply compare results obtained following the intervention with those obtained either earlier or without the intervention. These comparisons may be of the same group of people at various times (single-group designs) or of different groups.

Single-Group Designs

There are two types of single-group designs: pre-post designs and time series designs. An example of a pre-post design is seen every Sunday in newspaper advertisements for weight loss products. They invariably present a fuzzy "before" photo, followed by a vivid (and skinny) "after" shot. The reader scoffs at this gimmick. After all, there is no reason to be sure that the 200-pound loss was caused by the diet product. Maybe the model also had a tummy tuck or liposuction. Or maybe she would have lost the weight anyway, knowing that her photo would be put in the paper. And who knows whether she kept the weight off after the "after" photo was taken.

These responses illustrate the problems with the pre-post design. It does not eliminate other possible explanations for the changes observed. However dramatic the improvement may be, it may have occurred even without the program. Further, there is no way of knowing how long the improvement was sustained. To a limited extent, these problems are eliminated when a time series design is used.

While the pre-post design involves only two snapshots, the time series involves several, taken at key intervals. The savvy marketer of diet products might use this approach, offering annual photos of models—from 5 years before they bought the product to 5 years after their drastic weight loss. The photos taken before would establish their obese baselines and weaken the suggestion that they would have lost the weight anyway. The series of "after" shots would lead one to believe that the improvements were not temporary and might be expected to persist.

The time series design does strengthen an argument that change was due to participation in the program. But it does not conclusively rule out the possibility that caregivers would have shown improvement without the program. Suppose, for example, that the program was developed at the same time that Congress passed phenomenal improvements in the Medicare program. The decline in caregiver stress observed in program participants might be equally due to this historical event.

Comparison Groups

A group of caregivers who did not participate in training but who were monitored during the same period would help rule out this possible explanation. This comparison group might be drawn from a variety of sources. If the program maintains a waiting list, those on the list might be periodically surveyed. Caregivers who drop out of the program may serve as a comparison group. Caregivers can serve as their own comparison group if they are willing to wait to begin training.

While useful, a comparison group differs from a control group in one very important way: Its members may consistently differ from those in the treatment group. And these differences may explain the differences between groups observed after the program. For example, caregivers who drop out of training may be under greater stress than those who completed training. If they show no improvement over time, and the training participants do improve, it might be because of the different stress levels rather than because of the training. So the observed difference between the groups may not necessarily reveal a program outcome (treatment effect).

Consistent differences between comparison and treatment groups are problematic but not devastating to the evaluation effort. To the extent to which these differences can be measured, statistical procedures can be used to control for them. Instead of using a simple t-test to compare group scores, the evaluator may resort to multivariate techniques, such as MANOVA (Multivariate Analysis of Variance). If the observed treatment effect persists it is much more likely to be real. If it does not, the evaluation effort has revealed a potentially important relationship between the intervening variable (in this example, stress) and the outcome of treatment.

CLIENT SATISFACTION

The "smile-o-meter" approach to evaluation is held in some contempt by purists. Yet it is a wonderful source of qualitative data regarding how a program is perceived by the most important evaluators: its participants. Those who choose not to employ a more rigorous evaluation strategy will find client surveys both affordable and palatable.

A primary concern with client surveys is minimizing their "demand characteristics." This term refers to a human tendency to tell people what they want to hear. For example, even the most disgruntled participant probably will respond positively when the trainer corners him or her after a session to ask how the program is going. If program advocates are in need of testimonials about how wonderful the program is, they may exploit these demand characteristics, asking questions such as, "On a scale of 1 to 10, how much did you like this program?" The wording of this question tells the respondent exactly what the evaluator wants to hear: how very much he or she *liked* the program. The question is unlikely to elicit feedback about what the participant *did not* like about the program.

Demand characteristics can be minimized in several ways. First, those who conduct the training should not interview participants about their satisfaction. Second, participants may be given a form to complete that clearly disguises their identity. For example, in one program, participants are given an evaluation form at the end of the last session. They are asked to mail it in using a prepaid envelope addressed to the agency evaluator. A third way to reduce demand characteristics is to avoid using wording that will bias responses. Instead of asking how participants "liked" a program, evaluators might ask for the participants' opinions of the program.

Client surveys should address four things: (a) clients' general response to the program; (b) clients' impressions about how the program has or has not affected their behavior; (c) clients' assessment of program elements that were particularly useful; and (d) clients' assessment of program elements that were not particularly useful. The sample form at the end of this chapter includes questions that address each of these areas (see Table 3.3).

SELECTING MEASURES

Evaluation studies conducted to date have shown little or no improvement on global outcome measures (Barusch & Spaid, in press; Toseland & Zarit, 1989). But specific behavioral indicators often show considerable change. Because program goals are often broad, I do not recommend discarding global measures altogether. Instead, evaluators should combine them with specific measures that are directly related to program objectives. As outlined in Chapter 2, goals and objectives might include reducing caregiver distress, enhancing social support, facilitating behavioral change, supporting personal goal attainment, or reducing nursing home placements. The following sections describe available measures that have been used with each of these goals and objectives.

Measures of Caregiver Distress

Most research on caregiver distress relies on global self-report measures. The most widely used measure is a burden scale, developed by Zarit, Reever, and Bach-Peterson (1980). This is a 22-item inventory that focuses on subjective dimensions of burden, with statements such as "I feel guilty about my interactions with my spouse." Caregivers are asked to report their agreement or disagreement with each statement using a 5-point Likert scale, ranging from "strongly agree" (1) "to strongly disagree" (5).

Another approach to measuring caregiver burden was developed by Rhonda Montgomery and her colleagues (Montgomery, Gonyea, & Hooyman, 1985). This 22-item scale distinguishes between objective and subjective burden. Objective burden refers to "the extent of disruptions or changes in various aspects of the caregiver's life and household." Nine items were developed to measure objective burden (Montgomery & Borgatta, 1989). Subjective burden "reflects the caregiver's stress and nervousness related to her or his situation and the extent to which the caregiver feels manipulated by the demands of the care receiver" (Montgomery & Borgatta, 1989). The 13 questions used for measuring subjective burden were derived from those in the Zarit et al. (1980) inventory.

The Cost of Care Index represents a similar approach to measuring caregiver distress (Kosburg & Cairl, 1986). This 20-item scale measures four potential and actual costs of caring for an older person:

personal and social restrictions, physical and emotional health, problems with the care recipient, and economic costs. It also measures caregivers' values related to caring.

Another dimension of caregiver distress is measured by depression scales. Among these, the Beck Depression Inventory is most widely used. It contains 21 categories of symptoms and attitudes. There are four response choices for each category, indicating frequency of occurrence. Greater depression is indicated by higher scores (Gallagher, 1987). Another, self-report approach to measuring depression is the Brief Symptom Inventory (Derogatis & Spencer, 1982).

Depression is not the only form of distress experienced by caregivers. Hostility, anxiety, and resentment may be of concern; a caregiver may also experience more positive feelings, such as confidence, energy, and clarity of thought. Measures of these feelings are less well researched than depression measures.

The Bradburn Affect Balance Scale (BABS) is a 10-item scale designed to measure emotional well-being (Bradburn, 1969). The Profile of Mood States—Bipolar Version (POMS-B) shows promise for measurement of both positive and negative feelings experienced by caregivers (Gallagher, 1987). This adjective checklist is available through the Educational and Industrial Testing Services.

Measures of Social Support

Despite widespread recognition of its importance, we are not entirely sure what social support is. It may refer to the number of different people (both family and friends) who are available to provide assistance. Or it may describe the number of people to whom a caregiver feels close. Or it may reveal the amount of help and support a caregiver receives. Finally, social support may be measured as the extent to which a caregiver feels satisfied with his or her relationships with family and friends. A caregiver program may affect any, several, or all of these.

The challenge for the evaluator is to select a brief, reliable, and valid measure for the dimensions of social support the program is expected to influence. Several measures are available. The Lubben Social Network Scale (LSNS) measures four aspects of social support: the number of people with whom the person has contact; the number of people to whom the person feels close; the frequency of social contacts; and the availability of a confidant. This scale includes 10 questions, is easy to score, and seems to be a valid measure (Lubben, 1988).

Other measures address the amount and nature of the assistance received. The CSP project used an inventory developed by Robert Milardo (Milardo, 1983). This inventory focuses on emotional support, measuring both positive and negative social contacts. It lists 25 possible activities, such as "provided you with a place where you could get away for a while" or "criticized or showed frustration or anger at the way you were doing things." We asked caregivers to report how often someone performed each activity during the previous two months. Responses were coded using a 9-point scale ranging from "never" (0) to "once a day or more" (9). Two subscales were developed, measuring positive and aversive contacts. (See Barusch & Spaid, 1989, for more detail.) We also asked caregivers who usually performed each activity, to identify sources of support as well as strain.

Finally, two measures described by Mangen & Peterson (1982) offer an approach to gauging the caregivers' satisfaction with family and friends. These are called the "Family APGAR" and "Friend APGAR." Each contains five statements relating to satisfaction with various dimensions of relationships with family or friends. Respondents use a 3-point Likert scale to indicate agreement.

Notably absent in these scales is a measure of the help caregivers receive with specific tasks of caregiving. Evaluators interested in this dimension of support might adapt the "Extent of Caregiving" scale (Toseland et al., 1989a) described in the section "Measures of Caregiving Skills and Tasks" in this chapter.

Although global measures are attractive in their capacity to simplify information they have proven problematic in the evaluation of caregiver interventions. Published evaluation reports generally reveal little or no improvement using global measures. This may be because the measures are not sensitive to the specific changes that caregivers experience, or because of a tendency for caregivers to underreport their levels of stress. For this reason, evaluators who use these scales should combine them with more specific or personalized measures of change (Zarit & Toseland, 1989). These include measures of behavioral changes that may result from training as well as those that gauge the extent to which caregivers reach their goals for change.

Measures of Behavioral Change

Coping Measures

Measures of caregiver coping abilities use either checklists to evaluate the frequency with which caregivers use particular coping strategies (Pratt, Schmall, Wright, & Cleland, 1985) or an open-ended approach to describe how they cope with specific problems (Barusch, 1988). Each approach has advantages and disadvantages. Checklists are quickly administered and controlled. An open-ended approach yields an extensive understanding of caregivers' own perceptions of their coping responses, but is time-consuming and labor intensive.

The Family Crisis-Oriented Personal Evaluation Scales (F-COPES) uses 30 questions in a checklist format to evaluate the frequency with which individuals and families use eight possible coping strategies (McCubbin, Larsen, & Olson, 1981). These strategies include reframing, passivity, confidence in problem-solving abilities, and the use of five possible sources of social support: spiritual support, extended families, friends, neighbors, and community services (Olson et al., 1983). The F-COPES has been used successfully to evaluate the coping strategies used by family caregivers of Alzheimer's victims (Pratt et al., 1985).

A similar checklist was developed by Anne Jalowiec (Jalowiec, Murphy, & Powers, 1984). The Jalowiec Coping Scale consists of 40 coping behaviors. A 5-point Likert scale indicates how often a person used each behavior. Coping behaviors can be classified as problem-oriented and emotion-oriented. This scale has also been used successfully in research on caregivers (Wright, Lund, Caserta, & Pratt, in press).

A Coping Inventory developed by CSP uses an open-ended approach to describe coping responses. It presents 34 situations that might pose problems for the caregiver. Problem situations are divided into six major areas: care management, personal and psychological problems, interpersonal problems with spouse, interpersonal problems with others, financial problems, and other problems. If a caregiver reports experiencing a problem, the inventory provides an open-ended format for describing the coping response used. The caregiver then evaluates the effectiveness of each coping technique using a 5-point Likert scale ranging from "not at all effective" (1) to "completely effective" (5) at solving the problem. A coping effectiveness score can be computed for each of the six categories. This represents the average effectiveness rating assigned to problems in that category that the caregiver experienced (sum of effectiveness ratings/total number of problems experienced). An overall score can be computed in the same way.

Measures of Caregiving Skills and Tasks

It is likely that intervention will influence the nature of tasks performed by the caregiver. Ron Toseland has developed a measure of the "Extent of Caregiving," which might prove useful in this regard. This is a 27-item scale that lists specific tasks involved in caregiving, such as "help with bathing" or "supervise the taking of medications as prescribed." Caregivers are asked how often they have performed each task, using a scale from "never" (1) to "daily or more often" (5) (Toseland et al., 1989a). A summary score can be calculated or involvement in individual tasks compared.

Measures of Personal Goal Attainment

Goal Attainment Scaling (GAS) was initially used in the 1950s to evaluate mental health services. The technique responded to a need to avoid the inflexibility of standardized measures. Clients who entered the mental health system did not all share the same standard treatment goal. Similarly, caregivers differ in their reasons for participating in support programs. GAS offers a systematic approach to evaluating success in reaching individualized goals.

The self-care plan, described in Chapter 2, provided the basis for goal attainment scaling in the CSP project. The process can be accomplished in three steps:

1. Goal selection. Caregivers should be encouraged to identify personal goals that directly benefit them, not their loved ones. The number of goals chosen will vary from program to program but should not exceed five. Goals should be relevant (to the caregiver's well-being), specific, and measurable.

2. Statement of expected outcome. This step involves first stating the expected outcome, then describing outcomes that would be better or worse than expected. The expected outcome is what the caregiver thinks is most likely to happen. Others range from the worst possible case to the best possible case. An example is presented at the end of this chapter. These will form the behavioral anchors for a Likert scale that can be used to evaluate success.

3. Follow-up. Progress reports may be taken periodically. (In the CSP program caregivers reported weekly.) They also may be taken as part of posttests and long-term follow-up interviews.

GAS offers both specific and global measures of program outcome. Caregiver goals can be scrutinized individually or in groups, and a summary score can be calculated indicating the average success across goals. A sample GAS form is included as Table 3.4 at the end of this chapter. (See Kiresuk and Lund, 1978, for a more detailed description of GAS procedures.) A variation on the GAS theme was developed by Ronald Toseland (Toseland, Rossiter, & Labreque, 1989b), a measure called the "Pressing Problem Change Index." Care-givers were asked to identify pressing problems related to caregiving. A Likert scale was used after training to ask caregivers to evaluate the degree of change in each problem (Toseland et al., 1989b). This is similar to an approach described by Brahce (1983).

Another approach to goal attainment scaling was used by the CSP project. Self-care plans (described in Chapter 2) were used to help caregivers establish personal goals for the training. Caregivers then reported each week on their success in reaching those goals. When retained, caregivers' self-reports can be used in the evaluation process.

Measures of Nursing Home Placement

There is some (albeit limited) evidence that caregiver groups can affect use of nursing homes (Greene & Monahan, 1987; Montgomery, & Borgatta, 1989). Measuring placement is not entirely straightforward. Caregiver programs may increase nursing home utilization, even as they decrease permanent placement. Some caregivers who participate in programs are introduced to the possibility of using nursing homes for respite. Others use them temporarily following an acute health crisis. Among the CSP caregivers who did use nursing homes, only 43% saw the placement as permanent. So evaluators who monitor nursing home placement also should monitor the caregivers' reasons for placement and the expected duration of the stay. If long-term follow-up is possible, the number of days spent in a nursing home also might be obtained.

The frequency of nursing home placement is low, even among those caring for severely disabled patients. As a result, programs must be large to demonstrate a measurable change in the rate of placement. Smaller programs may consider using a proxy measure of likelihood of placement. For example, the CSP program asked caregivers to estimate the likelihood that they would use a nursing home within the following year. (Lund, Pett, & Caserta, 1987, also used this measure.) This can be done using a scale that ranges from 0% likelihood (this will never happen) to 100% likelihood (this will certainly happen). Caregivers' initial estimate was significantly associated with whether they did use a nursing home ($p < .05$), indicating the measure is valid (Barusch & Spaid, in press).

PROBLEMS IN EVALUATION

Those interested in conducting an evaluation need to be aware of some general problems that can reduce the value of evaluation findings. These include alternate explanations, demand characteristics, reactive effects of measurement, self-selection, and regression toward the mean (secular drift).

The problem of alternate explanations was discussed in the sections on evaluation design. Briefly, this refers to the possibility that some event or condition other than the training intervention is causing the changes observed in program participants. The number of alternate explanations can be minimized through effective use of quasi-experimental designs.

The demand characteristics involved in measuring client satisfaction were also discussed in the previous section. These referred to the natural human tendency to say what others want to hear. Sometimes this includes a tendency to say things that are socially acceptable. So, for example, an older man may be reluctant to describe the amount of stress he is experiencing because, especially for his cohort, it is not considered appropriate to complain. Researchers have been surprised by how low caregivers score on some measures of depression (Gallagher, Rose, Rivera, Lovett, & Thompson, 1989). They have concluded that some may underreport their depressive symptoms. This may be because they find the symptoms embarrassing or because they are reluctant to complain. At any rate, demand characteristics need to be minimized during data collection and taken into account when findings are interpreted.

Similar to demand characteristics are the reactive effects of measurement. Reactive effects are observed when the measurement itself influences the problem or situation under consideration. Sometimes just talking to someone about a problem or writing something about it can make the problem get a little better. This can be frustrating for those who have made the effort to secure a true control group, because the control group may improve just because of the pre-test! If both control group and treatment group show the same improvement it may be due to the reactive effects of measurement. Alternatively, thinking about a problem may lead a caregiver to realize how bad the problem really is. Awareness of the possible reactive effects of measurement will facilitate interpretation of findings.

Self-selection limits the extent to which evaluation findings can be applied to different groups of caregivers. That is, the caregivers who chose to participate in a particular program may be very different from those who might choose to participate in an alternate program. Further, they probably are very different from the caregivers who would not choose to participate in any program. This is an evaluation problem affecting generalizability of findings. It also may be an intervention problem, in that caregivers who are reluctant to participate are probably those most in need of assistance. This has been further discussed in Chapter 2.

Secular drift can be both a bane and a blessing. This refers to a tendency for people to become more average over time—at least on paper. That is, people who score exceptionally high on a scale at pretest tend to show lower scores at posttest despite what went on in the meantime. It is a statistical probability that does not really reflect human behavior. So, if the eligibility requirements for a program involve exceptionally high scores on a stress measure, evaluation of the program is likely to show improvement, if only because of secular drift. Conversely, caregivers who underreport their depression are likely to show higher levels at posttest. They are so close to the bottom of the scale that there is little room for improvement, while people at the top of a scale have no place to go but down. This can be a hidden blessing for programs designed for the high-risk caregiver and a problem for those whose participants score low on pretest measures. It is frustrating for those interested in precise description of treatment effects because it is impossible to distinguish secular drift from genuine changes.

GENERATING AND REPORTING RESULTS

Evaluation results should be generated continuously. That is, the data collected for both process and outcome evaluation should be periodically compiled and examined by program staff. Reports should include basic statistics, describing the characteristics of the people served, and giving averages and ranges on process and outcome measures. Statistical techniques are beyond the scope of this work. Those interested in computer-aided analysis will find the SPSS/PC Advanced Statistics Users Guide extremely helpful (Norusis, 1986). Those working manually will find that the *Computational Handbook of Statistics* (Bruning & Kintz, 1968) provides step-by-step instructions for computing most statistics.

I think reports of evaluation findings are most effective when they combine statistics with qualitative material describing program impact. Besides describing the average change in outcome measures, evaluators should consider including case histories that illustrate the story told by the figures. Readers vary in their approach to information. Some are moved by abstract illustrations, such as graphs and tables, which reveal program impact. Others prefer the "bottom line"—average improvement. Still others find a touching story most persuasive. Effective presentation of evaluation findings will appeal to all three types of readers.

At this stage it is vital that evaluators keep in mind that there is *no such thing as a negative evaluation*. This is true, not just for their personal well-being, but also for optimizing the potential contribution of their efforts. A program that shows no overall impact should not be viewed as a failure.

When confronted with findings of no benefit, the evaluator has several options. First, the evaluator might compare the program to others like it. The program might be doing as well as, if not better than others in the field. This is particularly true of group interventions with family caregivers. Many evaluation studies have shown no significant overall improvement, and others have shown little. Second, the evaluator might look at specific as opposed to global measures. In the absence of overall improvement, specific measures or individual items on global scales may show some improvement. Third, the evaluator might identify a target population that does benefit. The program may not produce benefits for the hypothetical "average" client, but surely it worked for someone! The evaluator might identify the characteristics of those who did benefit from the program. These can be used for targeting later program efforts. Fourth, the evaluator might look at specific components, rather than the whole program. Although the program as a whole showed no impact, specific components may have been successful. Given the appropriate evaluation design, it may be possible to distinguish program components and compare their effects. Finally, if all else fails, ask the clients. Caregiver interventions typically have very high client satisfaction (Barusch & Spaid, in press). Even if this was not included in the original evaluation design it may be added as a post-hoc approach.

Evaluators who strike out on these options will need to use the reframing techniques described in Chapter 1. Instead of setting out to demonstrate the impact of the program, they might view their task as teasing out the valuable lessons that have been learned. These might reflect specific areas of difficulty that need to be addressed in later efforts. Or, the evaluator might conclude that limited resources need to be directed elsewhere. Ultimately, these findings may be more useful than those originally sought.

RESOURCES

Measures:

Gallo, J. J., Reichel, W., & Andersen, L. (1988). *Handbook of geriatric assessment.* Rockville, MD: Aspen Publications.

Kane, R. A., & Kane, R. L. (1981). *Assessing the elderly: A practical guide to measurement.* Lexington, MA: Lexington Books.

Mangen, D. J., & Peterson, W. A. (1982). *Research instruments in social gerontology: Social roles and social participation* (Vol. 2). Minneapolis: University of Minnesota Press.

Evaluation Design:

Campbell, D. T., & Stanley, J. C. (1963). *Experimental and quasi-experimental designs for research.* Chicago: Rand McNally.

Rossi, P. H., & Freeman, H. E. (1985). *Evaluation: A systematic approach* (3rd ed.). Beverly Hills, CA: Sage.

Statistics (not computer aided):

Bruning, J. L., & Kintz, B. L. (1968). *Computational handbook of statistics*. Glenview, IL: Scott, Foresman.

Examples of Evaluation of Caregiver Support Projects:

Symposium: The effectiveness of caregiver groups [Special issue]. (1989). *The Gerontologist, 29*,4 (esp. 437-481).

Table 3.1

Caregiver Screening Form

(Completed upon entry into the program.)

I. Caregiver Characteristics

    A. Gender   M   F   B. Age_____

    C. Main occupation (when working)_____

    D. Employment status   Employed   Partially Retired   Retired

    E. Relation to care receiver_____

    F. Health status: How would you describe your health at this time?

                Poor   Fair   Good   Excellent

    Any major health problems? _____

II. Referral Source

    A. Where did you learn about the program?

        Word of mouth _____

        Media _____

        Agency _____

        Other _____

III. Caregiving Situation

    A. Patient's primary diagnosis_____

    B. How many hours do you spend assisting or supervising this person
        each day? _____

IV. Motivation

    A. What is the main reason why you chose to provide care to your_____?

Table 3.2

Session Report

(Completed by trainers at the end of each session.)

1. Who provided the training? _____

2. Participation:

Client's Name*	Present?	Accompanied?	Comments

3. General comments on the session: _____

_____

_____

*To save time, these names should be pre-printed for each session.

Table 3.3

Client Satisfaction Survey

(Completed after training or at follow-up.)

1. General Evaluation

   A. Please circle the number that best reflects your
       opinion of this training program:

1	2	3	4	5
Disliked very much— "A waste of time."	Disliked somewhat	Neutral, not sure	Liked somewhat	Liked very much— "I learned a lot!"

   B. If you had a friend who was a caregiver, would you recommend
       that he or she participate in this program?   Yes   No
       Why or why not?_____

2. Program Impact

   A. Has this program changed the way you feel about
       caregiving?   No   Yes
       If so, how? _____

   B. Will you do things differently as a result of
       participating in this program?   No   Yes
       If so, what? _____

3. Strong Program Components

   A. Do you use anything you learned now?   No   Yes
       If so, what?_____

       Or

       Will you use anything you learned in the future?   No   Yes
       If so, what? _____

4. Weak Program Components

   A. If we have to cut some things out of this program what should we cut?
       (Please circle those you think we might eliminate, and indicate
       your reasons.)
           [List training sessions or program components here.]

General Comments: We welcome any thoughts you would like to share
about this program._____

Table 3.4
Goal Attainment Follow-up
(Sample form.)

Goal Attainment Levels	First Goal	Second Goal
	Reduce commitments	Get help
a. Worst Possible Outcome (1)	Increase in number of hours spent doing church work	No change in the amount of respite provided by friends or family
b. Less than expected success (2)	No change in number of hours spent doing church work	A slight increase that is achieved at great cost
c. Expected outcome (3)	Reduce the number of hours from 10 to 7	A moderate increase (2 hrs per week) is made available on request
d. Better than expected success (4)	Reduce the number of hours to 5	A moderate increase is offered without request
e. Best possible outcome (5)	Reduce the number of hours to 3	Friends and family offer substantially more respite with no request made

Total change score: $\dfrac{\text{Goal 1 plus Goal 2}}{2}$

Part II

BACKGROUND MATERIAL FOR INSTRUCTORS AND CAREGIVERS

This part of the *Wellsprings* curriculum is designed for use by instructors and caregivers. It includes background material and exercises that can form the basis of a training program. Each chapter corresponds to a training session in the *Wellsprings* program, providing in-depth coverage of the topic under consideration. At the end of each chapter you will find training suggestions and recommended exercises. Training exercises are presented in detail in Appendix B. Instructors probably will be unable to present everything in the chapter in one 2-hour session. Instead, I suggest that you choose those topics that will be most useful to you, using the other material as background reference. Caregivers also may find this part of the book a useful resource.

Part II includes six chapters. Chapter 4 discusses physical aging and self-care through nutrition and exercise. Chapter 5 focuses on emotional needs and how they can be met to maintain a healthy relationship. Chapter 6 describes community resources, including both health care and social service providers, and discusses ways of accessing these resources. Chapter 7 addresses legal and financial concerns. Chapter 8 presents two key caregiving skills: medication management and maintaining home safety. Chapter 9 discusses grief and mourning.

Chapter 4

NORMAL AGING

Caregivers and those who work with them are constantly exposed to older people who suffer from major disabilities. This can affect personal attitudes toward aging, leading them to expect disease and disability in old age. But disease and disability are the exception, not the rule, in later years. The vast majority, 80 to 90% of older persons, are self-sufficient (Branch & Jette, 1983; Dawson, Hendershot, & Fulton, 1987). This self-sufficiency reflects adaptation to the normal physiological changes that occur with age.

Normal aging is an oxymoron, a contradiction in terms. There is no such thing as normal aging. As humans age, life hones them in unique ways. Child development specialists can predict with surprising accuracy the age at which an infant will learn a specific skill such as raising his head or turning over. Human infants are remarkably alike. Human 80-year-olds are remarkably different from one another.

Although there is really no such thing as normal aging, there are physical and behavioral changes that generally (but not always) occur in later years. It is important to understand these changes and the meaning an individual assigns to them.

EFFECTS OF AGING VERSUS EFFECTS OF DISEASE

Failure to distinguish so-called normal or common effects of aging from the effects of disease can lead to tragedy. It is tragic, for example, when an older woman suffering from a reversible condition spends her final years in a confused state. This happens all too often when family members, physicians, and other professionals mistakenly assume that confusion is a natural consequence of aging.

Natural consequences of aging have three general characteristics:

1. They are universal. They are experienced by everyone, or nearly everyone, who ages.

2. They are gradual. They tend to happen slowly and don't just appear overnight.

3. They are due to internal processes in the body. Often, these internal processes interact with environmental conditions.

In his seminal work, *The View from 80,* Malcolm Cowley (1982, p.3) describes some feelings that accompany the normal aging process.

> The new octogenarian feels as strong as ever when he is sitting back in a comfortable chair. He ruminates, he dreams, he remembers. He doesn't want to be disturbed by others. It seems to him that old age is only a costume assumed for those others; the true, the essential self is ageless. In a moment he will rise and go for a ramble in the woods, taking a gun along, or a fishing rod, if it is spring. Then he creaks to his feet, bending forward to keep his balance, and realizes that he will do nothing of the sort. The body and its surroundings have their messages for him, or only one message: "You are old."

The following sections describe age-related changes, including skeletal changes, changes in organ systems, and sensory changes. Most of these changes result in greater vulnerability, increasing the risk and consequences of disease and accidents.

Skeletal Changes

Most of us take our bones for granted. We view them as we do concrete in a building. Like concrete, our bones support our weight. But they also protect vital organs, allow freedom of movement, and provide stability. They also serve as a storage site for minerals. Through the continuing process of bone remodeling, calcium enters and leaves the body. Within the bones, our immune system operates, sending out cells to fight disease and infection.

Two normal changes can affect the skeletal system:

1. *Diminished bone mass and thinning of cartilage.* These can lead to reduced height, increased risk of fractures, stooped posture, and limited mobility. Extreme loss of bone mass results in osteoporosis. Joint stiffness and pain are usually caused by arthritis. Over 80% of older people have some "rheumatic complaint" (Boss & Seegmiller, 1981). Stiffness and pain also may be associated with bone cancer. Chronic recurrent bone pain merits medical attention.

2. *Reduced immunity.* The immune system within the bones becomes less efficient with age. It responds less quickly to invasion and takes longer to replenish the supply of protective cells.

Changes in Organ Systems

Heart and lungs. In general, age-related changes in the heart and lungs result in diminished efficiency and greater vulnerability. Two changes are observed in the heart: (a) The heart grows larger. (b) There is a decline in cardiac output. Under normal circumstances, this change is not noticeable. The older heart works as well as the younger heart, but it usually takes longer for the heart rate to return to normal after exercise.

Unlike the heart, which generally functions well in old age, older lungs show greater effects as years go by: (a) Air sacs become frayed and less efficient. (b) Lungs become stiff and susceptible to infection or pneumonia. In later years, a mild infection in the chest can be lethal.

Kidneys and bladder. The kidneys and bladder function to remove waste from our bodies. They also help to regulate fluid levels. They are subject to several important changes in old age: (a) kidneys become smaller, and (b) they filter less blood and are less efficient at removing waste. As a result of these changes, the kidneys regulate fluid levels less efficiently. So dehydration can be a major problem, especially when accompanied by diarrhea or fever. Medications also can build up in an older person. Dosage is a sensitive decision with an older patient. So it is important that medications be managed by a physician with experience and training in geriatric practice.

The bladder is also subject to changes. The bladder is less expandable and less sensitive. As a result, it gives less warning. This is especially true for women who have strained it during pregnancies. So urinary incontinence is not unusual in older women. This can be managed, and in some cases, corrected with biofeedback, medication, or surgery.

Gastrointestinal system. The gastrointestinal system includes everything that contributes to "food processing" in the body. It begins with the mouth and includes the esophagus, stomach, and intestines. Although the teeth of older people are often in poor condition, this is not the result of normal age-related changes. Other normal changes do affect the mouth: (a) less saliva is available and (b) the muscles of the esophagus are less efficient. This can make eating less enjoyable and more difficult. When coupled with isolation, these changes can produce malnutrition.

The stomach and intestines generally wear well in old age but the large intestine may present some problems. Constipation is one of the most common. With some encouragement from the media, today's elderly often worry unnecessarily about constipation. This may be because they were raised in an era when constipation was thought to be associated with "autointoxication"—a process by which, it was believed, waste was reabsorbed in the body, having some poisonous effect. Daily elimination was thought to be a necessity. A study conducted in 1972 found that 25% of elderly who believed themselves constipated, in fact, were not (Eastwood, 1972).

For those who genuinely suffer from constipation, regular use of laxatives is discouraged. Exercise and fiber in the diet generally produce good results. Loss of bowel control is common, although not necessarily normal in the 80s and 90s. This can be managed with enemas and suppositories or, in some cases, treated.

Nervous system. The human nervous system is made up of cells that, unlike other body cells, cannot be replaced. Over a life span, nerve cells are lost. This generally results in slower information processing and some inefficiency within the nervous system. It also produces some of the sensory changes associated with advanced age.

Sensory changes. Age brings with it several changes in our senses. These affect hearing, taste and smell, pain, and vision.

Hearing. Hearing often declines with age starting in the 50s and 60s. This is especially true of men. It usually involves (a) loss of higher frequencies and (b) difficulty understanding speech. Hearing loss can be due to gradual deterioration of the inner ear. It also can be due to build up of wax in the ear. Those suffering from hearing loss are more likely to become withdrawn and depressed. Many types of hearing loss can be corrected with hearing aids.

Taste and smell. Changes in the nervous system result in increased thresholds for taste and smell. Smell is an important component in appetite.

As their sense of smell diminishes, the elderly become more vulnerable to malnutrition. Also, body odors and bathroom odors can go undetected, and the elderly become less likely to detect spoiled food.

Pain. Nervous system changes also can raise the threshold for pain in old age. It becomes harder to detect painful sensations. Failure to detect heat can lead to tissue damage, for example, through scalding or burning.

Vision. Vision almost universally declines with age, but most older people have serviceable sight for life. Normal changes include (a) a general decrease in the accuracy of depth perception, (b) slower adaptation to changes in light, (c) increased sensitivity to glare, and (d) reduced night vision.

These changes can influence a person's daily life. Many older people choose not to drive or, lacking adequate night vision, may not drive at night. Homes that were safe can become hazardous (see Chapter 8 on home safety).

Three common conditions affect vision in old age: cataracts, glaucoma, and macular degeneration. Cataracts are the most common vision-related disability experienced by the elderly. A cataract makes the normally transparent lens of the eye opaque. This interferes with the passage of light and reduces visual acuity. Initially this is experienced as dimmed, blurred, or "misty" vision. People may need brighter light in which to read and complain of glare. Surgery is nearly always successful in relieving this condition.

Glaucoma develops slowly. When symptoms are noticed, permanent loss may have already occurred. Roughly one in every twenty people over 65 develop this condition. It is caused by increased pressure inside the eye and may produce eye aches, headaches, nausea, halos around lights, and loss of peripheral vision. Glaucoma can progress to total blindness. Everyone over 65 should have yearly eye exams to check for this condition. Many clinics and hospitals provide free examinations.

The macula is the central focusing area of the retina that enables us to make fine discrimination and identify detail. With macular degeneration, a person loses the central visual field. Peripheral vision remains intact. Macular degeneration is the fourth major cause of blindness in the United States, and the number one cause of serious visual deficiency among the elderly.

COGNITIVE AND BEHAVIORAL CHANGES IN OLD AGE

Mild Memory Impairment

Memory changes are not unusual as a person ages. Many older people experience what physicians call "benign senescent forgetfulness." These memory changes usually involve problems with registration and retrieval—that is, recording facts and getting them back out again. Fortunately, memory can be improved. A variety of mnemonic techniques are described in the books listed in the resource section of this chapter. Also, B. F. Skinner has written a delightful book entitled *Enjoy Old Age,* which presents several pointers on coping with mild memory impairment.

Some elderly suffer memory changes that are caused by reversible factors: malnutrition and dehydration, many medications, stress, boredom, depression, melancholy, lack of stimulation, hormonal changes, and general poor health. Those who experience subtle memory changes may become alarmed, worried that they signal irreversible dementia. They may want to consider the reversible causes listed above as possible explanations. It also may help to try some mnemonic techniques. Finally, if the concern persists, it may be helpful to seek medical advice.

Intelligence and Learning

Does intelligence decline with age? Can you teach an old dog new tricks? Answers to these questions are complex and controversial. Recent studies have shown that the average person's general intelligence increases with age, at least up to age 50, and that this increase in intelligence is maintained well into the 60s. This is particularly true of one type of intelligence called "crystallized intelligence." This refers to the mental abilities that depend on experience and on education in the broad sense including both formal schooling and the informal learning experiences of everyday life. It is a type of "common sense." Crystallized intelligence often shows a dramatic increase with age (Cunningham & Owens, 1983; Owens, 1966; Schaie & Strother, 1968).

Speed of information processing declines with age, as does motivation to perform meaningless tasks. So an older person may take longer to complete an examination or learn new material. This should be taken into account in training programs for older caregivers.

Personality Changes

A prevailing myth holds that people become more rigid and conservative in their later years. Personality change in old age is rare and typically associated with pathology. Habits may change and single aspects of a personality may become slightly exaggerated, but basic personality does not change dramatically with age.

Jung suggested that gender roles change with age. In his view, women become more masculine as they age and men more feminine. Research supports the notion that women often learn to be more assertive in their later years; and men, more nurturing (Hooyman & Kiyak, 1988). Rather than viewing older women as more masculine and older men as more feminine, it may be appropriate to view both as more androgynous.

Sleep

In later years, people tend to spend more time in bed and less time asleep. It is not unusual for an older person to nap during the day and to awake several times during the night. Unless the person feels tired during the day, these changes should be viewed as normal. Dramatic change in the sleep pattern might be an indication of problems.

Insomnia is a frequent response to anxiety and stress. In this situation, most physicians will discourage chronic use of sleep medication. Exercise is recommended for those who have mild difficulty falling asleep. The familiar glass of warm milk also may help induce sleep. For more suggestions on how to get to sleep, see Leonard Felder's book, *When a Loved One Is Ill: How to Take Better Care of Your Loved One, Your Family, and Yourself* (1990, p. 66-73).

Confusion

Many elderly people experience confusion at some point. Often it is minor. It should never be viewed as normal. The stress of caregiving can produce confusion as can a variety of other reversible conditions such as heart disease, pneumonia, kidney problems, a change in body temperature, a change in blood sugar, some medications (sleeping pills, tranquilizers, anti-depressants, and high blood pressure medication). More often than not, confusion is temporary. When it is severe and sudden, it should be treated as a medical emergency. It should never be neglected or viewed as a natural result of aging.

PHYSICAL SELF-CARE THROUGH NUTRITION AND EXERCISE

Nutrition

Age-related changes also affect our nutritional needs and our eating habits. With age, the number of calories needed each day is reduced. Yet our need for vital nutrients, such as protein, calcium, and many vitamins is greater than ever. So as we reduce our caloric intake it is important to optimize the nutritional value of the foods we eat. It is not unusual for older Americans to have diets that are deficient in essential nutrients including calcium, iron, and B-complex vitamins (Watson, 1985).

Further, common health problems can dictate new eating habits. High blood pressure requires reduced sodium intake. Heart problems call for eating less fat. Those suffering from diabetes will need to reduce their sugar intake. Drugs can also affect a person's metabolism, leading to deficiency of specific nutrients.

Recommendations about nutrition are often complicated and controversial. The *New American Eating Guide,* was prepared by the Center for Science in the Public Interest, and is recommended by Fallcreek and Mettler in *A Healthy Old Age* (1983). Another publication, *Nutrition and Your Health: Dietary Guidelines for Americans,* prepared by the U.S. Department of Agriculture (listed in "Resources" at the end of this chapter) is considered less controversial. Both might be used as references for further information on nutrition.

Most nutritionists and the Food and Drug Administration recommend that we sample from four basic food groups each day. These are listed below.

Meat: Two 6-ounce servings per day

Dairy: Two one-half cup servings per day (women may need more)

Fruit and vegetables: Four servings (variety is important)

Grains and breads: Four servings per day

Caregivers might find it helpful to think of the past 24 hours and consider whether their diet is meeting the needs of their body.

Millions of dollars are spent each year on advertising for the latest diet or latest appetite control measure. Instead, small behavioral changes will go far toward improving health and nutrition. Caregivers should be encouraged to identify times of day or situations in which they tend to overeat or eat inappropriately and use their self-care plans to avoid doing so. They also may want to consider making some minor changes in their diet to accommodate their bodies' responses to stress. This might involve taking a supplement of B vitamins and a good multi-vitamin and mineral supplement. Also beneficial is substituting herbs for salt. See Fallcreek and Mettler (1983) for suggestions and recipes that will support good nutrition.

Exercise

Unfortunately, the first principle of self-care that most caregivers abandon is a regular exercise program. The benefits of exercise spill over into better nutrition habits and mental health.

The ideal exercise program has three components:

1. Flexibility: Every exercise session should begin and end with stretching to improve flexibility and avoid injury.

2. Strength: Strength can be a key to independence enabling us to lift and move our bodies at will. Exercises that are weight-bearing contribute to muscle and bone strength. Isometrics are also helpful. In general, anything that provides resistance to the muscle is helpful. Strengthening exercises help prevent osteoporosis and muscle weakness.

3. Endurance: Exercise for endurance contributes to the fitness of the pulmonary and cardiovascular systems. This type of exercise is most often neglected by older persons, yet it is the most valuable for weight control, depression, and insomnia. Exercises that use large muscles in continuous movement such as swimming, walking, and bicycling are recommended. These should be done three or more times per week for at least 20 minutes. Endurance exercise should be preceded by a 10- to 15-minute warm-up and followed by a 10- to 15-minute cool-down period.

Caregivers may want to consider investing in a device that would enable them to get aerobic exercise without leaving home. This device might also be used by the care receiver. Many older Americans are purchasing treadmills. Other alternatives include stationary bicycles, rowing machines, and small trampolines. Some exercise videos are now tailored to older people, offering low-impact aerobic workouts and gentle stretching.

There are many good sources for information about exercise for the elderly. One particularly valuable source is a pamphlet from the American Association of Retired Persons (AARP) entitled, "Pep Up Your Life: A Fitness Book for Seniors" (see "Resources" at the end of this chapter).

Caregivers (like most of us) are inclined to use their lack of exercise as another reason to feel guilty. Instead they can be encouraged to view exercise as self-care, and select the type of exercise that will be most enjoyable to them. If they like to talk with neighbors, a fast walk to a friend's house may be in order. Window shoppers might enjoy walking through the nearby mall. Many malls open early for this purpose. Television fans may want to put a treadmill in front of the TV.

SUGGESTIONS FOR TRAINERS

When using the content in this chapter as part of a training program, the following objectives are relevant:

1. Help participants understand the difference between normal aging and the effects of disease
2. Provide specific information about physiological changes with age
3. Provide information about cognitive and behavioral changes that come with age
4. Introduce nutrition and exercise as tools for self-care

It is often helpful to invite a nutritionist to present material in this area. Trainers will also find good handouts in Fallcreek and Mettler (1983), listed in the resource section of this chapter.

RESOURCES

Books:

Basic exercises for people over sixty and moderate exercises for people over sixty. Available for $1.00 from National Association for Human Development, 1750 Pennsylvania Ave., N.W., Washington, DC 20006.

Fallcreek, S., & Mettler, M. (1983). A healthy old age: A sourcebook for health promotion with older adults. *Journal of Gerontological Social Work, 6,* 2/3.

Help yourself to good health. Produced by the National Institute on Aging, available through PFIZER Pharmaceuticals, 230 Brighton Road, Clifton, NJ 07012-1498.

A national directory of physical fitness programs for older adults. Available for $4.00 from North County Community College Press, Saranac Lake, NY 12983.

Pep up your life: A fitness book for seniors. Available through the American Association for Retired Persons (AARP), 1909 K Street, N.W., Washington, DC 20049.

Skinner, B. F., & Vaughan, M. E. (1983). *Enjoy old age: Living fully in your later years.* New York: Warner Books.

Tomb, D. A. (1984). *Growing old: A handbook for you and your aging parents.* Harrison, VA: R. R. Donnelley & Sons.

Memory Books:

Higbee, K. (1988). *Understanding your memory.* Englewood Cliffs, NJ: Prentice-Hall.

Lapp, D. (1987). *Don't forget: Easy exercises for a better memory at any age.* New York: McGraw-Hill.

West, R. (1985). *Memory fitness over forty.* Gainesville, FL: Triad.

Nutrition Books:

Center for Science in the Public Interest. *The New American Eating Guide.* 1501 16th St., N.W., Washington, DC 20036, (202) 332-9110.

Composition of Foods (No. 8, covers all food groups). Superintendent of Documents, GPO Bookstore, 1961 Stout St., Room 117, Denver, CO 80294. (303) 844-3964. Cost: $7.00.

National Clearinghouse on Aging, SCAN Social Gerontology Resource Center. *Nutrition/Nutrition Programs Bibliography,* including references on nutrition and aging. P.O. Box 231, Silver Spring, MD 20907.

Nutrition and Your Health: Dietary Guidelines for Americans (U.S. Home and Garden Bulletin No. 232, 1990) (3rd ed.). Available through your local county cooperative extension office.

Chapter 5

HEALTHY RELATIONSHIPS

There is no simple technique for maintaining a healthy relationship while coping with serious illness. Yet the relationship is central to the well-being of both caregiver and care receiver. To provide support for that relationship, this chapter addresses two concerns: emotional needs and communication. The ongoing crisis presented by a disease interferes with both aspects of a relationship. First, the physical demands of caregiving may leave little time or energy to address emotional needs. Second, the fear and anxiety generated by illness can impair open communication. Finally, in relationships that have been distant, the intimacy of caregiving can introduce new pressures and challenge existing communication patterns.

EMOTIONAL NEEDS

In a caregiving situation, the physical needs of the care receiver are often the dominant concern. These needs are important and must be met on a day-to-day basis. But the patient's physical needs can be met by someone other than a caregiver. Organizations such as home-health care services and Meals on Wheels have been established in many areas to help meet these needs.

Emotional needs are more exclusive. In the face of mounting physical needs, the emotional needs of both patient and caregiver are frequently overlooked to the detriment of both. Emotional needs should be viewed as necessities of life, on par with physical needs. Some common emotional needs include a sense of self-worth, control over decisions, a confidant, and a sense of productivity.

Sense of Self-Worth/Capacity for Self-Love

Our sense of self-worth (or self-esteem) is our emotional assessment of our personal value. It is our answer to the question "What good am I, anyway?" Self-esteem is crucial in determining our response to the many challenges presented in a lifetime. Researchers find that people with high self-esteem more readily adapt to traumas, such as widowhood, than do those with low self-esteem (Lund et al., 1985/1986). Self-worth is closely linked to self-love. The importance of self-love for caregivers is reflected in a statement Erich Fromm made in *The Art of Loving:* "'Love thy neighbor as thyself!' implies that respect for one's own integrity and uniqueness, love and understanding of one's own self, cannot be separated from respect and love and understanding for another individual" (1956, p. 49).

Our sense of self-worth is maintained through both internal and external validation. Internal validation refers to our "self-talk," the valuative statements we make to ourselves. Negative statements such as, "I'm such a dummy! Why didn't I remember her name? I met her yesterday!" diminish our self-worth. Positive statements, on the other hand, can support our sense of worth: "Boy, I sure look good today! No one would know I only had three hours of sleep!" External validation comes from the significant others in our lives, including family members, friends, and colleagues. Like self-talk, external validation can either support or diminish our sense of self-worth. Some friends serve as constant reminders of our flaws, others as loyal cheerleaders (see the descriptions of supportive and destructive people in Chapter 9). Those of us who are particularly self-critical may discount the positive validation we get from others. When receiving a compliment, instead of accepting it with thanks, we discount it, saying, "Oh, this little thing! It's nothing! I'm just doing what anyone would do!" Besides the negative impact this has on the person who offers a compliment, it deprives us of a much-needed boost to our sense of self-worth.

People vary, both in the amount of validation they need and in the supportive feedback they find meaningful. Those who care a great deal about their appearance may draw great support from a compliment about a dress; for others this would provide little satisfaction.

Both caregiver and care receiver often experience blows to their sense of self-worth. Caregivers who have given up jobs to provide care often come to realize how much their self-esteem was related to their work role. Loss of that role may mean loss of the external validation provided through work. Also, caregivers who have relied on the patient for validation may find that support unavailable as the care receiver focuses on his or her illness. The isolation associated with caregiving can jeopardize self-worth by depriving the caregiver of external validation.

Illness can be a serious blow to the care receiver's sense of self-worth. This is particularly true when disease forces people to abandon meaningful roles and activities. Those who took pride in their physical appearance and abilities may find the ravages of disease particularly damaging to their sense of self-worth.

Both caregivers and care receivers can deliberately enhance their sense of self-worth through three approaches:

1. *Maximize all positive validation and defuse or ignore negative feedback.* Instead of discounting compliments, caregivers and care receivers can practice hearing and accepting them. Then they can turn discounting skills to any criticism or negative feedback both internal and external. As Melba Colgrove pointed out, "There is no need to give negative thoughts about yourself prime time status" (1981, p. 24).

2. *Caregiver and care receiver might agree to exchange three sincere compliments each day.* Compliments not given during the day might become due and payable at bedtime. If the care receiver is cognitively impaired the caregiver may need to find another person to join in the agreement.

3. *Give affirmations.* Affirmations are positive, loving statements a person uses periodically throughout the day, such as "I, Betty, am a warm, loving, competent person." Some people put the statements on their mirrors or carry them in their wallets. They provide handy substitutes when self-critical thoughts surface and, some believe, through constant repetition they become true! Norman Vincent Peale wrote extensively about affirmations in his 1956 work *The Power of Positive Thinking.* The interested reader will find more material on this topic in the resource section of this chapter.

Control

We all have a strong desire to control our environments. Control has several forms: ability to decide the outcome or what will happen, ability to predict events, and ability to determine how we will respond to events (Baltes & Baltes, 1986). Illness frequently takes away some control. It may present caregiver and care receiver with outcomes they cannot determine and events they cannot predict. By draining their emotional reserves, it can even impair their ability to respond to events in the way they would like. Loss of control is frightening. The general goal of control-focused intervention is to optimize the forms of control available to a person and minimize the negative emotional and cognitive effects of loss of control.

For the care receiver loss of control can be especially problematic, as it extends to physical capacities and bodily functions. The situation is worsened when those around the sick person confuse loss of physical control with loss of decision-making ability. This is seen when doctors and other professionals talk to the caregiver about the patient in the patient's presence. It is not unusual in a doctor's office for the care receiver to be excluded from discussions about his or her care. In a sense, the patient is treated like a child or, worse, a nonperson.

Some people who are treated like children begin to act like children. Rather than verbally protesting loss of control they make a statement by acting out their frustration, for example, by throwing food on the floor. After repeated experiences with loss of control, a person may sink into a state of "learned helplessness." In this state of passivity, initially described by Martin Seligman (1975), a person simply abandons efforts to control his or her environment and seems incapable of learning.

Albert Bandura (1977) described the sense of "self-efficacy"—the converse of learned helplessness—as the belief that one can control the environment and effect change. To support care receivers' sense of self-efficacy it is important to optimize their control of the environment. This means involving patients in decisions that affect them and the people they care about. It also means giving choices in day-to-day decisions such as what to wear or eat.

The same principle applies to caregivers. Confronted with so many things they cannot control, caregivers need to identify how they can exercise control. When faced with uncontrollable events and conditions, caregivers can focus on gently controlling their response to and interpretations of these situations. This does not suggest discounting or suppressing unpleasant or unacceptable emotions. The rage or sorrow needs to be accepted and experienced. But caregivers can control their "self-talk," or interpretation of events. Techniques such as reframing (see Chapter 1) and relaxation (see Appendix B) can be used to optimize this form of control.

Confidant

Most people benefit from having a close friend or confidant. This is someone who will listen, accept and care, and refrain from giving unwanted advice. Access to one or two confidants may be especially important in late life (Bell, 1981; Strain & Chappell, 1982).

A person's ability to find a confidant will depend on his or her lifelong style of friendship. Mathews (1986) identified three friendship patterns:

1. *Independent:* People using this style form associations with those they come across, avoiding strong emotional ties. These people are likely to report that their spouse is their only confidant.
2. *Discerning:* People who use this friendship make commitments to a small group of close friends. As these people grow older, the small group dwindles, leaving them isolated.
3. *Acquisitive:* People who use this style form close friendships with new people throughout life. By acquiring new friends, they have more contacts and confidants when they are older.

It is unlikely that caregivers or care receivers will change their basic approach to friendships; however, it is useful to recognize the pattern that prevails, and acknowledge the important role of confidants. Besides providing positive validation, confidants can reduce stress by allowing a person to express (ventilate) his or her feelings. A confidant also can help normalize feelings, providing assurance that a person is not "crazy" but rather experiencing natural reactions to a difficult situation. A lifelong confidant is especially well qualified to remark on certain habits of thought or emotion that might be affecting a person's reactions.

Confronted with the pressures of caregiving and the limitations of illness, both caregiver and care receiver can become isolated from their confidants. Caregivers often lose their lifelong confidants. This may be particularly true of men, who tend to have less extensive friendship networks than women. Even those with many friendships are likely to neglect friendships when confronting serious illness.

Caregiver interventions can help reduce this isolation by acknowledging the importance of confidants and encouraging caregivers to maintain friendships. It is unlikely that people who have been "independents" all their lives will suddenly open to intimate friendships when involved in caregiving. Still, acquaintances that arise in caregiver groups sometimes provide a safe substitute for lifelong confidants.

Productivity

Productivity has two aspects. The first, "internal" aspect depends on our personal values, our sense of meaning. This aspect of productivity is supported by activities that we find personally rewarding and we believe are valuable. The second, "external" aspect of productivity depends on what other people value or need. We can feel useful while engaging in activities that we do not find particularly rewarding but that other people need. A retired scientist might support the internal aspect of productivity by continuing in some aspects of his lifelong research after retirement. The external aspect might be supported by more mundane tasks such as setting the table for a family dinner.

Caregivers generally feel productive and needed. Care receivers often do not. Yet both have the same need. Even care receivers who are severely regressed need to feel productive. Patients can be encouraged, for example, to help with simple tasks, such as peeling potatoes, clipping weeds, or cleaning silver. Although it may take them twice as long to do something, it is important to acknowledge and support their efforts.

Respite

Respite is an interval of rest or relief. Respite provides a temporary escape or a "break" from the pressures of the immediate situation; an opportunity to replenish depleted energy reserves. It is not synonymous with the use of formal respite services, such as those provided by a senior companion or adult day care center. Respite services may provide an opportunity for respite, but caregivers usually do not recognize their need for respite and are reluctant to use substitute care for a real break. Instead, most caregivers spend their respite time taking care of errands and other pressing matters.

Just as the availability of respite care does not ensure true respite, unavailability of substitute care does not preclude it. Caregivers can use times their help is not needed (when the patient is resting, for example) to take respite. Respite may take many forms: watching daily soap operas, reading truly trashy novels, listening to music, going for a walk, or socializing with a friend. The relaxation exercises in Appendix B can provide a feeling of temporary respite. It is helpful for both caregiver and care receiver to have a special place for respite, a "safe harbor." Just as most people need nurturing social contacts, most people need nurturing places. These are places of safety and rejuvenation. For some a safe harbor may be a city bench, where strangers passing by know nothing about the pressures at home and pigeons are grateful for any scrap of bread. For others it might be a neighbor's kitchen or a local recreation center. Care receivers might find safety in a day care facility or a neighborhood park. Sometimes reaching into memories and using visualization can take people to a safe harbor (see the visualization exercises in Appendix B.)

A few moments spent in a safe harbor can ease stress. If one is not available, caregivers might create a special and comfortable place in the corner of a room, where stressful thoughts are not allowed to intrude. Pictures, wallpaper, furniture and fabrics can be used to establish an atmosphere of ease.

BALANCING PHYSICAL AND EMOTIONAL NEEDS

To maintain a healthy relationship between caregiver and care receiver, it is important that both focus on the other person, not on the illness. The illness presents physical needs that must be met. Because of their immediacy these physical needs often distract everyone involved from the emotional issues. Sometimes the caregiver will find it easier to do for the patient than to be with the patient. If this is the case, it suggests that emotional needs have been neglected and must be given higher priority. A healthy relationship will depend on both the caregiver's and care receiver's ability to focus on the other person and not on the disease.

Caregivers can be encouraged to address emotional needs in any kind of training format. The checklist at the end of this chapter can be used as a homework assignment or an in-class exercise. Essentially it asks, "To what degree does the caregiver allow each need to be met for both him- or herself and the care receiver?" While filling out the checklist, the caregiver should be encouraged to identify innovative ways of meeting these needs.

COMMUNICATION

Because human communication is so complex it can easily go awry. The sending and receipt of messages is a constant process. Messages are rarely simple. Usually they have at least two layers of meaning. On the surface a message means exactly what the words spoken convey. At a deeper level a message conveys the emotion the speaker experiences while speaking. At even deeper levels, messages can convey the speaker's socioeconomic status, family history or even philosophy. They also can convey the speaker's assumptions about the listener, showing whether the listener is seen as friend or foe, informed or naive, and so on. The words chosen to send a message represent the tip of the iceberg that is the message. Under the surface, the deeper layers of meaning are conveyed by nonverbal (and sometimes invisible) cues.

Communication can go awry at either the sending or the receiving end. Problems with sending are usually the result of incongruence. That is when the layers of a message do not agree. Often verbal and nonverbal messages have different meanings. For example, the words "I love you" when delivered in a gentle tone provide a congruent message. But when the underlying tone of voice is angry and the speaker is pushing the listener out the door the message becomes confusing at best. When messages are incongruent it is usually the nonverbal message that is received.

Sometimes incongruence results not from disagreement among the layers of a message, but from inappropriate emphasis on the unimportant aspects of the message. The key aspect of a message may be hidden by camouflaging words. This often happens when the speaker is embarrassed or ambivalent about the primary message. For example, an 80-year-old woman who calls her daughter at work several times a day to discuss trivial details may be using the details as camouflage for her underlying concern that the daughter's job will make her unavailable.

Communication problems also can occur at the listening end of the process. Listening can be contaminated by inaccurate assumptions or by interference. In the above example, the daughter may be so overwhelmed by responding to the superficial messages that she does not perceive her mother's fear. This may be because the daughter has always assumed that her mother was independent and not "needy." Or, because the underlying important message was hidden in all the interference (discussion of trivial details).

Misunderstandings are so common that we often just accept or ignore them. Sometimes we decide that the message just was not worth the effort. When we do this we devalue both ourselves and the other person. It is important to correct misunderstandings as soon as possible. As a rule, if a person still remembers the misunderstanding it is probably worth bringing it up. As we practice at correcting misunderstandings we usually learn to avoid miscommunication.

The pressures of coping with serious illness increase the likelihood of miscommunication in part because little energy or time is available for avoiding or clarifying misunderstandings. Illness also brings a series of new roles and expectations to a relationship. With these new roles comes a greater need for strong communication. Caregivers and care receivers need to talk about these new roles and negotiate how they will handle decision making and problem solving. If communication has not been good in the past, this discussion will be particularly difficult. Caregivers can often benefit from learning specific communication skills.

Exercises that support direct, assertive communication are presented in Appendix B. Two techniques that enhance communication are "I-statements" and active listening. One is a sending skill, the other a receiving skill.

1. *"I-statements."* When communicating about emotionally charged issues concentrate on describing feelings using "I" rather than "you." With I-statements the speaker assumes responsibility for his or her feelings and communicates them in a way that is less threatening to the listener. For example, rather than saying, "You make me so angry when you do this stupid thing!" (which is heard as "You are so stupid!"), use an I-statement, such as "I feel angry when you refuse to take your medication."

2. *Active listening.* This technique involves nonverbal and verbal responses that let a person know that he or she is being heard. Nonverbal responses include eye contact, head nodding, even touching. Verbal responses range from the ubiquitous "uh-huh" to paraphrasing what the person has just said. Paraphrasing might sound like this: "Are you saying that you are frustrated by the way the doctor treats you?" Lead phrases such as, "Are you saying . . . ," "Here's what I understand . . . ," or "It sounds like . . ." are often used in paraphrasing.

When a person is ill for a long time he or she often begins to feel like others are not listening. (This is often a legitimate feeling; see the "Control" section above.) Caregivers can help patients by using active listening.

The interested reader will find more material on communication in Adler & Towne's *Looking Out, Looking In, Interpersonal Communication* (1975).

Healthy relationships do not necessarily meet all a person's emotional needs. Caregivers often must go outside the caregiving relationship to meet these needs. It is important that everyone involved in the caregiving ecosystem acknowledge the emotional needs of both caregiver and care receiver. Often caregivers must educate those around them to respect emotional needs just as they do physical needs. Communication is central to this process, just as it is central to maintaining a healthy relationship. Families that have not used direct, open communication are unlikely to do so suddenly when confronted with serious illness. But, even in the most uncommunicative families, intervention efforts can empower the caregiver to use new communication skills to support his or her self-care efforts.

SUGGESTIONS FOR TRAINERS

When leading a training session on emotional relationships, the following objectives apply:

1. help caregivers reevaluate the quality of their relationship with the patient, recognizing not only the physical but the emotional needs of both;

2. continue the process of self-care by the presentation of stress management and communication skills;

3. encourage participants to take active steps toward fulfilling their emotional needs and those of their patient; and

4. support caregivers' self-love by practicing the art of receiving compliments.

The goal in this session is to underscore the reality and urgency of emotional needs for both the caregiver and the care recipient and to remind caregivers that failure to respond to the emotional needs of the sick spouse often intensifies the demand to meet physical needs.

Following a discussion of emotional needs, two communication skills might be introduced: negative assertion and negative inquiry. Participants should practice these skills in pairs, then report to the group. As an alternative, leaders may want to focus on receiving and delivering compliments as a communication skill in support of self-worth (see Table 5.1)

RESOURCES

Books

Peale, N. V. (1956). *The power of positive thinking.* Englewood Cliffs, NJ: Prentice-Hall.

Adler, R., & Towne, N. (1989). *Looking out, looking in, interpersonal communication* (6th ed.). Troy, MO: Holt, Rinehart, & Winston.

Table 5.1
Emotional Needs Checklist

To what degree are you allowing these emotional needs to be met for yourself and for your loved one?

Yours (Caregiver)   *Ill Person (Care Receiver)*

ENCOURAGING A SENSE OF SELF-WORTH
(I have done something worthwhile in my life.)

1   2   3   4   5   1   2   3   4   5

HAVING CONTROL
(I can make decisions, I have the right to fail.)

1   2   3   4   5   1   2   3   4   5

HAVING AT LEAST ONE CLOSE FRIEND BESIDES EACH OTHER
(a confidant with whom I can share my innermost thoughts.)

1   2   3   4   5   1   2   3   4   5

HAVING A SENSE OF PURPOSE
TWO ASPECTS: INTERIOR AND EXTERIOR
(I have activities I find rewarding and meaningful and
I have activities other people find useful.)

1   2   3   4   5   1   2   3   4   5

FINDING RESPITE
(a time of relief in a place that is safe)

1   2   3   4   5   1   2   3   4   5

Chapter 6

TAPPING COMMUNITY RESOURCES

Self-care requires effective use of community resources. When CSP caregivers were asked what advice they would give to others in similar situations their first response was, "Get help; use services." This chapter describes professionals and services available in many communities. It also presents suggestions for selecting and working with a provider. It is divided into two sections: a guide to health professionals and a guide to social service providers.

A GUIDE TO HEALTH PROFESSIONALS

This section describes health care professionals who are likely to work with older patients and suggests how to choose and work with a provider. Recent years have seen tremendous growth in the knowledge and services designed to meet our health care needs. As a result the number of specialties within the field has increased to the point where few lay people know the names of the different providers, let alone what they do.

Health Care Providers

The confusing array of professionals serving older patients includes physicians, nurses, rehabilitation specialists, and pharmacists. The following sections describe the activities of these health professionals.

Physicians

For routine medical care most adults use a primary care physician, either an internist or a family practitioner. The primary care physician usually serves as the "front line" of health care, dealing with routine health problems, monitoring overall health, and detecting the warning signs of special problems that require referral. For older people, the front-line provider might be a specialist in geriatric medicine.

Women should have an established relationship with an obstetrician/gynecologist (OB/GYN). The OB/GYN diagnoses and treats diseases and disorders of women's genital, urinary, and rectal organs. Women beyond childbearing age may prefer to work with a doctor who specializes in gynecology as opposed to obstetrics (pregnancy and delivery). Annual visits to the OB/GYN will ensure early diagnosis of problems such as cancer of the cervix and breast.

For special medical care it is not unusual to be referred to a surgeon, cardiologist, oncologist, or psychiatrist. Surgeons usually specialize in particular parts of the body. For example, a thoracic surgeon treats diseases of the heart, lungs, chest wall, diaphragm, and major blood vessels. Cardiologists deal with heart problems. Oncologists specialize in the detection and treatment of cancer. They typically do not perform surgery, but typically use needle biopsies for diagnosis and chemotherapy for treatment. Psychiatrists diagnose and treat mental, emotional, and behavioral disorders. They often specialize in the treatment of a particular age group. For example, a geriatric psychiatrist works with older adults. Some specialize in the treatment of specific problems, such as anxiety, alcoholism, or depression (see Table 6.1).

Nurses

Typically nurses work under the supervision of a physician, either in an office, a health care setting, or a patient's home. There are several classifications of nurses, depending on level of training.

1. *Nurse practitioner or clinical nurse specialist.* Nurse practitioners (NPs) are highly trained nurses. They provide general medical care, patient assessment, and treatment. They may perform physical exams, order, interpret and evaluate diagnostic tests, maintain patient records, and, under a physician's supervision, recommend some treatment.

Table 6.1
Physician Specialties

Anesthesiologist: Administers anesthetics during surgical, obstetrical and other medical procedures.

Audiologist: Specializes in diagnostic evaluation of hearing, and treatment of auditory problems.

Allergist—immunologist: Diagnoses and treats diseases and conditions with allergic or immunological causes, including bronchial asthma, dermatological disorders, connective tissue syndromes, transplantation reactions, and auto-immunity.

Cardiologist: Treats diseases of the heart and its functions. Examines patients, prescribes medications, recommends dietary and work activity programs. Refers patient to surgeon specializing in cardiac cases when need for corrective surgery is indicated.

Colon And Rectal Surgeon: Deals with disorders of the intestinal tract, rectum, anal canal, and perianal areas that are amenable to surgical treatment.

Dermatologist: Diagnoses and treats diseases of human skin (acute and chronic).

Family Practitioner: Provides comprehensive medical services for members of family, regardless of age or sex, on a continuing basis. Examines patients; administers or prescribes treatments or medications; and promotes health by advising patients concerning diet, hygiene and methods for prevention of disease.

Gastroenterologist: Deals with diseases of the esophagus, stomach, small and large intestines, liver, pancreas, and gallbladder.

General Practitioner: Attends to a variety of medical cases in general practice. Orders or executes various tests and examinations and diagnoses conditions. Administers or prescribes treatments and drugs. Inoculates and vaccinates patients, and promotes health by advising patients concerning diet, hygiene, and methods for prevention of disease.

Geriatric Physician: Deals with the medical problems of the elderly.

Geropsychiatrist: Specializes in mental, emotional, and behavioral disorders of the elderly.

Gynecologist: Diagnoses and treats diseases and disorders of female genital, urinary, and rectal organs.

Hematologist: Diagnoses and treats diseases of the blood.

Internist: Diagnoses and treats diseases and injuries of human internal organs.

Nephrologist: Diagnoses and treats diseases of the kidney.

Neurologist: Diagnoses and treats organic diseases and disorders of the nervous system, but does not do surgery.

Neurosurgeon: A surgeon who evaluates and operates on lesions of the brain, spinal cord, and peripheral nerves.

Oncologist: Specializes in diagnosis and treatment of cancer through needle biopsy and chemotherapy.

Ophthalmologist: Diagnoses and treats diseases and injuries of eyes.

Otolaryngologist: Diagnoses and treats diseases of the ear, nose, and throat.

Pathologist: Prepares diagnosis based on lab tests of tissue samples.

Podiatrist: Diagnoses and treats diseases and deformities of the human foot.

(continued)

Table 6.1 Continued

Pulmonologist: Diagnoses and treats patients with diseases of the lungs.

Radiologist: Diagnoses and treats disease of the body using X-rays and other substances. Compares X-ray findings with other examinations and tests. Treats benign and malignant internal and external growths by exposure to radiation.

Rheumatologist: Diagnoses and treats a wide variety of diseases of the joints, soft tissues, and blood vessels.

Thoracic Surgeon: Operatively treats diseases and injuries of the heart, lungs, chest wall, diaphragm, and great vessels.

Urologist: Diagnoses and treats diseases and injuries to the kidney, ureters, bladder, and urethra. In males they also treat disorders of the prostrate and genitals.

2. *Private duty nurses.* Private nurses contract independently to provide care, usually in the home of one patient. According to physicians' instructions and the patient's condition they administer medications, treatment, dressings, and other services.

3. *Registered nurses (RNs) and licensed practical nurses (LPNs).* RNs and LPNs provide general care for people in hospitals, private homes, clinics, and nursing homes.

4. *Community health nurses.* These nurses instruct individuals and families on health promotion and disease prevention. They may work with individuals to identify health care needs and develop a plan for meeting those needs.

Rehabilitation Specialists

Rehabilitation specialists help people who are recovering from a stroke or other acute medical crisis to "relearn" independent living skills. These specialists include the following types:

1. *Physical therapists (PTs)* help people to rebuild muscle strength and maintain joint flexibility. They work in a variety of settings: hospitals, nursing homes, home-health agencies, and private practice. They may help patients to perform basic tasks, such as walking.

2. *Occupational therapists (OTs)* help patients learn how to perform complex activities, such as feeding, grooming, and bathing themselves.

3. *Speech therapists* help patients recover their ability to communicate. This may include use of communication devices, such as aids to amplify voices and communication boards, as well as instructing the patient in use of his or her voice and overcoming difficulties that impede speech.

Pharmacists

Besides dispensing medications, pharmacists can answer questions about side effects, possible drug interactions, refills, proper use of a medication, and screening for drug allergies. Many pharmacists will help a patient identify a less expensive generic alternative to a drug prescribed by a physician. Often a pharmacist is the best source of information about over-the-counter medications. (See Chapter 8 for a discussion of medication management.)

Choosing a Physician

Many (maybe most) people do not systematically shop for a physician. We tend to accept the first alternative offered, then do our best to live with the situation. Selecting a physician is an important decision. It merits time and effort.

The first step in choosing a doctor is compiling a list of possible candidates. Friends may not be the best source of recommendations because they may be like us in temperament but unlike us in medical needs and approach to health care. The perfect doctor for one person may be absolutely wrong for another. A better source would be hospitals and health professionals in the area. Many hospitals offer a referral service for those seeking a physician. Naturally, this service would only refer patients to physicians who are affiliated with the host hospital. In some communities, the local medical association may be a source of recommendations.

In some areas, especially rural areas, a shortage of physicians leaves consumers with few options from which to choose. When there is choice, the considerations presented below will help a person to narrow the list to those who merit an introductory interview. Many physicians will meet with potential patients free of charge as long as they will not be expected to provide medical care or opinions. Ask for a free interview. Before "doctor shopping" it is important to know whether there will be a charge for the introductory meeting.

Considerations

A variety of factors will influence the selection of a particular physician. Each person will weigh them differently. Some will value an excellent diagnostician over warmth and friendliness. Others may place office decor above convenience. It is important to think about these considerations before selecting a doctor. This will maximize the chances of a good match.

Professional credentials. Physicians can be either "board-certified" or "board-eligible." Those who are board-certified have taken and passed a qualifying examination in their area of specialty. Those who are board-eligible have met the requirements (education, residency training, and so forth) to take the examination but have not taken or have not passed the exam. It is also helpful to know how long the physician has been in practice, what medical school he or she attended, and where the physician served as a resident or a fellow.

Structure of the practice. Some doctors practice alone, others are in a group practice. A group practice has the advantage in that it offers the skills of other professionals (sometimes nurses and therapists as well as doctors) and usually provides for better coverage when the office is closed.

Hospital affiliation. Some health care experts feel that a doctor's hospital affiliation should be one of the most important considerations. The patient needs to be satisfied with the hospital's reputation. Often hospitals that are affiliated with universities are excellent choices.

Financial arrangements. Financial concerns need to be carefully explored. Patients should find out about these issues:

1. *Doctors' fees.* Fees may vary according to the nature of the medical problem.
2. *How payment is handled.* Must bills be paid at the time of the appointment? Does the doctor offer an installment plan for major medical bills?
3. *Insurance coverage.* Some insurance companies require that policyholders use certain physicians. It is important to be aware of these restrictions.
4. *Insurance claim forms.* Some doctors will submit claims directly; others require that patients provide payment and then submit the claims themselves.

Also, it is important that Medicare recipients learn whether the doctor "accepts assignment." Some physicians charge patients additional fees above what Medicare will pay (see Chapter 7, "Legal & Financial Concerns"). Those using Medicaid need to be sure the doctor accepts Medicaid and will bill directly.

Convenience. Location of the doctor's office and availability of parking can be critical for patients with mobility problems. Off-hour availability is another factor. It is important to know how to reach the doctor when the office is closed. Waiting is one of the most demoralizing aspects of physician care. It is helpful to know how far in advance you might need to schedule a routine appointment and how soon you can schedule an urgent appointment. It is also useful to know how much time you are likely to spend in the waiting room.

During the initial visit you will get some idea of the usual wait. It may not hurt to ask the receptionist or physician whether the first wait was typical. Sometimes it is worthwhile to ask to be the first or second appointment of the day to minimize waiting room time. This is particularly true if the patient finds the waiting room a depressing place.

Convenience needs to be weighed against other considerations. While it is probably not as critical as a doctor's professional credentials it can set the tone for the health care experience.

Personal factors. The physician's "medical philosophy"—his or her beliefs about health and illness—should be compatible with those of the patient. For example, some doctors take life-style and emotional well-being into account in their understanding of illness. Others prefer to narrow their consideration to identifying specific microbes. Some doctors take an aggressive approach to treatment, using medication and recommending surgery more quickly than others. Others are more conservative, waiting to see how a patient's condition develops. These views will affect the treatment options presented. They also may reflect religious or cultural values.

Other personal factors that are related to the physician's medical philosophy are his or her willingness to use support programs and encourage patient involvement. For example, some oncologists make active use of support groups and teaching programs while others do not. Similarly, some physicians encourage patients to be actively involved in decision making and others do not.

Patients vary in their preference for active involvement. Some like to take an active role in their care, others prefer to be directed by the doctor. Older patients tend to be more likely than younger patients to want to place themselves completely in the doctor's hands. They are more likely to want doctors to make decisions for them and to think it is a poor idea to suggest alternate treatments (Beisecker, 1988). It does not matter what the preference is. What is most important is the compatibility of patient and physician.

Ultimately, trust and communication are the essentials of a successful relationship with a physician. It is absolutely critical that the patient trust his or her physician and that the physician communicate effectively.

Working with a Physician

With the selection of the best available provider, a patient begins what probably will become a long-term working relationship. Two dimensions of this relationship are communication and decision making.

Communication

Regardless of age, patients tend to assume a passive role in communicating with a physician (Beisecker, 1988). This is consistent with a tendency among older adults to view the physician as an authority figure who is above reproach.

The context of doctor-patient communication supports patient passivity. After waiting for what seems like ages to see the doctor, a patient is ushered into the examining room by a member of the support staff. Here the patient waits again, but there are fewer distractions. In isolation the patient can ponder his or her vulnerability. Finally, the physician arrives, clad in the traditional uniform of authority, with an air of urgency. The physician is clearly rushed for time and may be surprised that the patient has not yet disrobed. The message conveyed is often "This is a very important professional. You are lucky to have a chance to see him or her. The doctor does not have much time for talk so it is time to get down to the physical exam."

Patients who wish to take greater control of the interaction should arrive at the office equipped to ignore or diffuse these messages. Here are some possible approaches.

1. Promise yourself that you will not take your clothes off until you have talked with the doctor about what will happen during the exam.
2. Consider bringing a companion. Be sure to pick someone who will be on your side, regardless. Sometimes a companion will reduce the patient's control by forming a coalition with the physician (Beisecker, 1989).
3. Confront hidden messages directly, using phrases like "You seem so rushed. Are you sure you have time to work with me today?"
4. Bring a list of questions and take notes. In the rush and confusion it is easy to forget important matters that you want addressed.

5. Remember you have a right to ask questions. If the physician seems threatened by your questions point out that you want to go to bed at night without nagging doubts. Your doctor may need assurance of your trust. Sometimes if a physician responds as though he or she is personally threatened, it may be best to look for another doctor.

6. Remind yourself that the doctor is working for you, a medical consumer as opposed to a client (Reeder, 1972). This places you in a more active (and more responsible) position in relation to the physician.

7. Check to be sure that what you say is understood and you understand what you have been told. In communicating with the physician you need to be aware that he or she may have several distractions: fatigue, worry over the last or next patient, or concern about being far behind schedule, to name a few. It may take considerable effort to compete with these distractions and get your message across.

8. Learn about prescribed medications—how to take them, intended effects, and possible side effects (see Chapter 8 for additional material on medications).

Decision Making

Regardless of the extent of patient involvement in decisions, it is important to understand the factors that are taken into account when making a treatment decision. These typically include:

- Possible consequences of no action
- Possible side-effects of treatment
- Known efficacy of the treatment proposed

By actively questioning a physician about each of these factors a patient will have enough information to understand and participate in the decision-making process. Patients also need to ensure that the physician is aware of any unique considerations, such as the patient's attitude toward treatment, problems with compliance, secondary conditions, and financial resources.

Second opinions. Sometimes it is appropriate to seek a second medical opinion. This is true:

- When elective surgery is recommended.
- When a second opinion is required by medical insurance.
- When the primary physician has not answered questions to the patient's satisfaction.
- When the patient feels uneasy about a decision.

Getting a second opinion is the patient's privilege. The doctor should not object. If the doctor is a member of a group practice it is helpful to seek the second opinion from a doctor outside that group.

Alternative Health Providers

Caregivers should be aware of alternative health providers for two reasons. First they may offer a useful option for coping with a medical problem. Second, some charlatans use these titles and can do serious harm. This section discusses three alternative providers: chiropractors, acupuncturists, and naturopathic physicians.

Chiropractors

Chiropractic physicians are primarily concerned with the spine and how its interplay with the nervous system affects body functions. They often treat problems associated with the neck, back, and the joints. Emphasis is placed on correcting structural disorders of the spinal column and adjacent tissues. They use a wide range of techniques for diagnosis and treatment, including analysis of posture and spinal column, X-rays, and some laboratory procedures. Treatment usually involves manipulation, and may include nutritional counseling and other approaches. Chiropractors must have a minimum of two years in college and four years of chiropractic instruction. They are licensed in all U.S. states and territories and their services are covered by many health insurance companies.

Acupuncturists

With its roots in ancient Chinese healing practices, acupuncture aims to affect a person's energy level and with it the functioning of internal organs, by either stimulating or depressing their action. Although it primarily involves inserting needles at key points in the skin, the practice of acupuncture can include a range of activities, from taking pulses, to application of heated materials, consideration of life-style, and the use of herbs. It is most widely used in the control of pain but has been used to address many complaints.

Acupuncturists are licensed to practice independently in 21 states. Those who are licensed in these states have completed their training in an approved school and have passed a national exam. In states where the practice is unregulated, consumers need to be careful because anyone can use the title. The National Commission for the Certification of Acupuncturists maintains a list of qualified practitioners and can refer people to a qualified acupuncturist in their area (see the "Resources" section of this chapter for the address and phone number of the NCCA).

Naturopathic Physicians

Naturopathic medicine is an eclectic healing profession, using natural substances and techniques to promote health and healing. Naturopaths use a wide range of techniques, including herbal medicine, nutrition, manipulation, massage, and counseling. They do not use synthetic drugs or perform major surgery. The practice of naturopathic medicine is less wide spread than either chiropractic treatment or acupuncture.

Naturopaths are licensed in eight states: Alaska, Arizona, Connecticut, Florida, Hawaii, Oregon, Utah, and Washington; the District of Columbia; and five provinces in Canada. This means that in these areas only those who complete four years of graduate training after receiving their bachelor's degree and who pass state and national licensing exams can use the title. Where naturopaths are not licensed the title is unprotected, which means that a person can call him- or herself a naturopath with no legitimate credentials. In these areas the consumer must be extremely cautious in selecting a provider. The American Association of Naturopathic Physicians (AANP) provides a referral service to help individuals locate a qualified practitioner (see "Resources" for the phone number and address of the AANP). About 90 insurance carriers in the United States and Canada cover naturopathic treatments.

A GUIDE TO SOCIAL SERVICES

Most caregivers make use of health care providers but are reluctant to use social services, associating them with welfare. They might need to be reminded that these services are often provided through tax dollars and that they have paid taxes for many years, earning the right to use them. Caregivers often find it difficult to negotiate the maze of services. This section describes the services available in many communities and offers suggestions for making the most of them.

Area Agency on Aging Services

Area Agencies on Aging (AAAs) were established throughout the United States in accordance with the Older Americans Act of 1965. Their function is to support independent living for the elderly by providing a wide range of services. They may be housed in different types of agencies such as universities, local government agencies, state government, or even the United Way. Most AAAs do not provide services themselves, instead, they purchase them from private organizations. Services provided through AAAs include mandated services, which must be made available, and optional services, which may or may not be provided in any given area.

Mandated Services

AAAs are required to spend "an adequate proportion" of their yearly allocation for mandated services. These include "access" services, which help people reach the services they need; in-home services; and legal services.

Access Services

Outreach/information and referral. The information and referral phone number is usually listed in the government agency section of the phone book. By calling this number, the caregiver can receive information about services available in his or her community.

Transportation. Most AAAs provide transportation only for specific purposes. Usually, transportation is provided for any medical need. This might involve doctors' appointments or visiting a spouse in a nursing home. Some agencies also provide transportation to senior citizen centers and other services such as grocery runs and transportation to entertainment.

In-Home Services

Homemaker services. Homemakers come into the home to help with light housekeeping tasks, such as vacuuming, dusting, and dishwashing. Usually this service is available once a week.

Home health aides. A home health aide provides personal care and some health-related care. He or she may help with bathing or checking blood pressure, for example, but would not change a catheter.

Visiting or telephone reassurance. This service is usually staffed by volunteers, who contact older homebound people periodically to see how they are doing and identify any pressing needs.

Chore services. Chore services help with home maintenance, performing tasks such as clearing rain gutters, minor home repairs, and shoveling snow.

Legal Services

A lawyer is provided to people with limited incomes. The lawyer can help with things like wills and guardianships but usually will not help with civil suits or criminal matters.

Other Services

Other services provided by AAAs include nutrition programs, both congregate meals in senior centers and home-delivered meals; socialization programs, such as the activities available in senior centers and other volunteer programs; protective programs to prevent or remedy elder abuse and neglect; employment programs for seniors; and case management services.

Nutrition Programs

Congregate meals. Many communities provide meals in senior centers and other settings. Usually this is lunch, and there is a brief program after the meal. These meals are available to anyone who wants them. Sometimes a small donation is requested.

Home-delivered meals (Meals on Wheels). The Meals on Wheels program provides home-delivered meals. Unlike congregate meals, eligibility is restricted. In most areas, a physician must certify that a person is unable to prepare meals. Generally, the demand for this program exceeds supply. It also has a suggested donation, usually a nominal amount. The drivers of Meals on Wheels can be wonderful resource people. Usually the same driver delivers the meals each day. At the same time, the driver can check on how the person is doing and find out about any medical emergency that might require attention.

Socialization Programs

Senior Companion. The Senior Companion Program provides employment for low-income seniors. Senior Companions help homebound elderly, usually by providing respite for the caregiver. They are trained and provided with a small stipend for their services.

Senior center activities. Senior centers provide a wide range of activities, including arts and crafts, discussion of current events, dancing, and other social activities. Many centers also offer adult day care.

Foster Grandparents. The Foster Grandparent Program was established to provide meaningful activities for those over 65. Foster Grandparents work with children and people with special needs in a variety of settings including schools, nurseries, Headstart programs, and adolescent treatment centers.

Retired Senior Volunteer Program (RSVP). The Retired Senior Volunteer Program provides opportunities for meaningful activity. These volunteers provide services in diverse settings such as hospitals and libraries. The program provides recognition and insurance for these volunteers and covers some expenses.

Protective Services

Many areas have adult protective services. Staff of these programs investigate reports of elder abuse and neglect and intervene on behalf of the victim. Intervention may take the form of family counseling or guardianship proceedings. Sometimes the AAA will become the legal guardian.

Employment Services

Senior employment programs provide training and subsidies for people over 55 who are seeking employment. Most are federally funded, operating under the Job Training Partnership Act. Some of these programs also have job-development components, with staff who work with corporations and organizations to identify jobs for seniors.

Case Management Services

Case managers help keep a person at home or prevent nursing home placement by arranging for supportive services and monitoring the client's needs. Eligibility is usually based on income and need. The case manager is authorized to purchase services such as home-health care, housekeeping, and nursing care. The case manager also might be trained to manage family crises and conflicts and to help caregivers mobilize support from informal sources such as neighbors and friends. In many communities, private case managers are available to help those who do not qualify for AAA services. They can usually be found by asking for a referral from the local AAA.

Adult Day Care

There are two types of adult day care facilities. The first provides primarily social activity and supervision. The second operates on a medical model providing nursing care and some assistance with medical management. Both provide supervised care to patients during the day. Adult day care centers provide respite for caregivers and can be a safe harbor for the care receiver. They may be freestanding or part of a nursing home facility. A directory listing 847 centers is available through the National Council on Aging (see this chapter's resource section).

Hospice Services

Hospice care is provided to help patients live comfortably until they die and to help the family live with them as they are dying. It involves both medical care and social services, and may be provided in the home or in a hospital. The hospice team is usually made up of volunteers, social workers, and nurses. If the patient is to remain at home, this team will train caregivers to provide personal care and some medical care. They also offer emotional support to both patient and family. Hospice care can be paid for through Medicare (see Chapter 7).

The array of social services includes both public and private providers. These providers go by a variety of names, and may be housed in a wide range of institutional settings. Caregivers often find negotiating this maze of service providers a frustrating experience. Case managers can help in some areas, but usually caregivers, patients, and other family members must develop the skills needed for accessing services themselves. The following section addresses how to work with social service providers.

Working with Social Service Providers

Physicians use white coats and stethoscopes as symbols of authority, social service providers use regulations and paperwork. Caregivers can find these just as intimidating and even more frustrating. Getting effective service from a social service provider can require persistence and assertiveness. It is important not to accept the first "no" from a social service provider. Even later "no's" should be viewed with skepticism. Some of the communication techniques presented in Appendix B can help access services.

Before contacting an agency it helps to spend some time thinking about the problem situation and what might be done to address it. Caregivers may want to write down a clear description of the problem and what they would like the agency to do. It also helps to have all the facts together. These will vary, but often include the following:

- The household income and assets
- The potential client's age
- The nature of the potential client's diagnosis and when it was made
- The potential client's functional level (What activities is he or she unable to perform?)
- The availability of family and friends as resources
- The time you could come in for an appointment

It is rare to find the right person—even the right agency—on the first contact. So it is best to begin the search by phone rather than in person. Probably the first person you talk to will give the name and number of someone else who "might" or "should" be able to help. This second person is closer, but not quite right . . . and so begins the famous "runaround." It is important not to let this process be too frustrating.

To cope with the runaround, write down the name and title of each person you talk to, the date of the call, and what he or she told you. Then, with each successive phone call, give that information to the person you call. Say, for example, "Betty Jones, the intake worker at information and referral, suggested that you might be able to help me find an adult day care center for my father." Whenever someone tells you he or she cannot help, ask for the name of someone who might be able to.

If someone tries to refer you back to a person you have already talked to, read your notes and explain what happened in the previous conversation. Then ask for a different name. If you get stuck with someone who should be able to help but cannot or will not, ask to speak with the person's supervisor. If that does not work, call the person who gave you the name and tell him or her what happened. Ask for a different name or advice for working with the uncooperative person.

Because you may need to call someone back for more help it is best to begin the search early in the week. Mid-morning on Monday is probably the best time. By doing it as quickly as possible (without an intervening weekend) you increase the likelihood that the person will emember the earlier conversation. Be aware that most public mployees are not available during the lunch hour.

If you are unable to find the right person by phone, go back to the st of people you have talked to and find the name of the one who vas most helpful. Call him or her back and ask for an appointment to et more help in solving this problem. A face-to-face contact is much 1ore powerful than a phone call. The person will probably spend 1ore time thinking about your situation if he or she anticipates seeing ou. It may be helpful to take a companion to this meeting—someone vho will support your efforts to get help and provide emotional upport. Keep a log of your efforts to find help. Later, it may be used n a letter to policymakers about problems in the system.

Caregivers may need to become experts in government regulations. Vhen confronted with an uncooperative public agency it is helpful to now what the service is supposed to be doing and how complaints bout it should be handled. It also may be helpful to know where the gency gets its money. Private agencies may be subject to licensing equirements. In this case they will be regulated by a government .gency. Caregivers who are dissatisfied with the services provided by . private agency may want to complain to the regulating authority.

Ultimately, caregivers who are not satisfied with the social services vailable in their areas will find it productive to translate their rustration into advocacy efforts. This not only discharges anger but nay even improve the situation for themselves and others. Staff of ublic agencies are usually glad to provide a list of names, addresses nd phone numbers of key policymakers. The American Association f Retired Persons (AARP) is another resource for those interested in dvocacy.

Choosing to Use a Nursing Home

Contrary to worldwide stereotypes, Americans do not "warehouse" heir elderly in nursing homes. Caregivers make heroic efforts to .void placing a loved one in a nursing home. Yet for some, nursing 1ome care is the best alternative.

Once the decision to find a nursing home has been made, caregivers vill begin to look for the best one available. To the extent possible, the •atient should be encouraged to participate in the selection process. "wo pamphlets can help. The first, "The Right Place at the Right "ime: A Guide to Long-term Care Choices," is available through

AARP. The second, "The Hardest Choice: Selecting a Nursing Home for an Alzheimer's Patient," is provided by the American Health Assistance Foundation. (See "Resources" at the end of this chapter for addresses.)

Once a caregiver has identified a nursing home it is helpful to make several personal visits to observe the way the facility operates. These are some questions to consider.

1. How is the morale of the staff? Do staff members appear to enjoy their jobs. If so, that enjoyment will translate into better patient care.

2. What is the staff turnover rate? In many nursing homes the aids who work with residents leave their jobs frequently. These departures can be confusing and unpleasant for residents.

3. Will family members be allowed and encouraged to participate in care?

4. What kind of personal touches are there in patients' rooms? One nursing home has a sign in each room that tells visitors and staff what the patient likes to be called, the names and residences of family members, and the patient's hobbies and previous employment.

5. Are cognitively impaired patients cared for in a separate unit? Often those who are not cognitively impaired find it demoralizing to live with severely regressed patients. Further, if the patient is cognitively impaired, it may be helpful to know the extent to which restraints and tranquilizing drugs are used to control patient behavior. These forms of patient control should not be used for the convenience of staff.

6. Do patients participate in the management and policies of the home? Is there a resident council, for example, that meets regularly with management?

7. What are the transfer policies? Some nursing homes require that patients be transferred if their money runs out.

8. How are resident complaints resolved? Even the best homes have complaints. There should be an established procedure for working through these.

9. What hidden costs should be anticipated? It will be important to understand what is included in the daily rate and what is not. Often there are extra charges for rehabilitation services, wheelchairs, dental care, and incontinent care.

Caregivers also should investigate the home's reputation by talking to professionals in the community. These include the nursing home ombudsman, who can be reached through the AAA, and the patient's physician. Caregivers also may request copies of the latest report by the state licensing inspector as well as the state survey that nursing homes prepare annually for Medicare and Medicaid.

Remember that the contract signed on admission is legally binding. It may be advisable to have a lawyer review it and suggest revisions on the caregiver's behalf.

Once a home has been selected and the placement completed, caregivers need to prepare themselves for the strong emotional reactions they are likely to experience, as well as those of their family members and friends.

They are likely to feel guilty. It is also not unusual for family members, even distant ones, to be harshly critical of the decision. The patient, too, may protest. Many nursing homes have family support groups to help caregivers work through this transition.

It may be helpful for caregivers to view placement as an opportunity to focus on the emotional aspects of their relationship with the patient, using visits as times for reminiscence and closeness. Further, many caregivers choose to perform tasks after the patient is in a nursing home. For example, a caregiver may continue to shampoo the patient's hair, feed him or her meals, or do the laundry.

Nursing home placement does not end the caregiving experience. Instead, it relieves the caregiver from some responsibility for physical care, freeing time and energy for self-care and emotional contact with the patient.

SUGGESTIONS FOR TRAINERS

This session can be used to meet the following objectives:

1. identify existing community resources;
2. increase caregivers' awareness of the skills needed to access those resources;
3. develop and introduce the assertive skill sometimes called "broken record" (see Appendix B) that can be necessary to obtain services; and
4. make initial steps toward "politicizing" caregivers—introducing advocacy as a constructive use of frustration.

By this session, many participants will have progressed from expression of their frustrations with taking care of a sick spouse to identification of needs for services. There is, however, a serious gap between recognition of needs and taking the first step to obtain services. Resistance to using public services can be addressed in a friendly, loving confrontation that will move caregivers to take a small step toward accessing services. Every community has a unique service delivery system and this session should provide detailed information about specific community services. Some services are universal, such as those provided through the Older Americans Act, though they may be identified by different names. Information and referral is a required service. I suggest that leaders first contact their community's information and referral outlet.

Guest speakers might be used to acquaint participants with local resources. If possible, guest speakers should come from public-sector agencies. Those who represent private agencies may be more interested in selling their service than providing an overview of available services. Possible topics guest speakers might address include the following.

1. Selecting a nursing home, day care, or home health agency
2. Programs offered at the local senior center
3. Low-cost mental health and counseling outlets
4. Housing options
5. Health care clinics that specialize in geriatric medicine

These services are of little value to the caregiver who is unable to access them. Assertiveness, perseverance, and other skills must be nurtured during this session. Assertiveness should be discussed and a related technique such as the broken record may prove helpful. As a homework assignment, participants are asked to contact one service provider and report back on what the service does.

RESOURCES

Pamphlets

"The right place at the right time: A guide to long-term care choices." Available through Health Advocacy Services, American Association of Retired Persons, 1909 K Street, N.W., Washington, DC 20049. (202) 728-4888

"The hardest choice: Selecting a nursing home for an Alzheimer's patient." Available through Alzheimer's Disease Research, American Health Assistance Foundation, 15825 Shady Grove Road, Suite 140, Rockville, MD 20850. (800) 227-7998

"Directory of adult day care in America." National Council on Aging, 600 Maryland Ave., S.W., West Wing 100, Washington, DC 20024 (ask for order no. 2022). (800) 424-9046

Books

Rossi, T. (1987). *Step by step: How to actively ensure the best possible care for your aging relative.* New York: Warner.

Manning, D. (1985). *The nursing home dilemma: How to make one of life's toughest decisions.* San Francisco: Harper & Row.

Organizations

National Commission for the Certification of Acupuncturists
1424 16th Street, N.W., Suite 105
Washington, DC 20036
(202) 232-1404

American Association of Naturopathic Physicians
2800 East Madison Street
Seattle, WA 98112
(206) 323-7610

American Association of Retired Persons
Health Advocacy Services
1909 K Street, N.W.
Washington, DC 20049
(202) 728-4888

Chapter 7

LEGAL AND FINANCIAL CONCERNS

Caregivers can help take care of themselves and those for whom they care by understanding the legal and financial resources available to them. Public programs, such as Medicare and Medicaid, provide vital assistance in helping to cover the high cost of health care. "Medigap" insurance policies purchased from private insurance companies pay some costs that Medicare does not. Voluntary legal devices such as the durable power of attorney and living wills can enable us to guide our destiny during incapacity. If we become unable to handle our own affairs and have not left plans, court actions such as guardianships or conservatorships may be initiated in our interest.

This chapter offers an overview of some laws that are relevant to older Americans and legal aspects of providing care. It is not meant to substitute for expert legal advice. Laws can change. This is particularly true of the laws governing Medicare and Medicaid programs, and the amounts of premiums, deductibles, and copayments under these programs are adjusted annually. The specific information presented is current as of this writing (1991).

MEDICAL INSURANCE

Medicare

Medicare is the federal health insurance program designed to provide partial coverage for many necessary medical expenses. It was established by Congress in 1965 as Title XVIII of the Social Security Act. Unlike Medicaid, entitlement to Medicare benefits is not based on an individual's need. Instead, Medicare eligibility is based on eligibility for Social Security retirement or disability benefits. People who are over 65 years of age who are not eligible for Social Security (a very small percentage) may purchase Medicare.

Medicare benefits are provided through two separate programs, Part A and Part B. Part A of Medicare covers many hospital, skilled nursing home and home health services and some hospice services. Part B partially pays for doctors, therapists, ambulance, and diagnostic services as well as prostheses, medical equipment, and certain other medical services and supplies.

Enrollment in Medicare is normally handled through the Social Security office. Application for retirement benefits automatically triggers the Medicare application process as well. Part A (hospital) coverage is provided without charge. Unless the beneficiary notifies Social Security that he or she does not want Part B (outpatient) coverage, the monthly premium is automatically deducted from each Social Security check. Those who do not sign up for Part B when they enroll in Medicare may do so during a general enrollment period, held from January 1 through March 31 each year.

The Health Care Financing Administration (HCFA) is the agency within the Department of Health and Human Services that has responsibility for the Medicare program. HCFA contracts with private insurance companies (Medicare intermediaries) throughout the country to process and pay the Medicare claims. In Utah, for example, Blue Cross and Blue Shield handle Medicare claims.

Part A: Hospital Insurance

Medicare covers 90 days of hospital services in a single benefit period or "spell of illness," supplemented by 60 additional "lifetime reserve" days, each of which can be used only once and is not replaceable. A "spell of illness" starts when a patient is admitted to the hospital for at least a 3-day period of care and continues until 60 consecutive days after the person has left the hospital. The average length of a hospital stay by a Medicare beneficiary is much shorter than the days of coverage available. So, although Medicare does not cover more than 90 days in a benefit period, in reality few beneficiaries ever use their lifetime reserve days. A new benefit period begins once a Medicare beneficiary is out of the hospital or skilled nursing facility for 60 consecutive days.

Medicare does not cover all the costs of hospital care. On admission, the patient must pay the in-patient hospital deductible, which is currently $628. Medicare then covers most hospital costs for days 1 through 60. After the 60th day of hospitalization, a daily "copayment" is required. For each day in the hospital from day 60 through 90, the beneficiary must pay $157. After 90 days in a benefit period, a beneficiary must use the lifetime reserve days each of which has a copayment of $314.

Many Medicare beneficiaries buy private supplemental health insurance policies to cover these copayments.

The hospital benefit under Part A covers the following: room and meal charges, routine nursing services, drugs provided for use in the hospital, equipment and medical appliances, inpatient physical therapy, and most other hospital charges. It does not cover luxury items and extraordinary services such as private duty nursing services, private rooms (unless they are medically necessary), and the telephone and television charges. Medicare only covers "necessary" medical care, that is, those items and services determined by a physician as necessary. Services of physicians are (even in the hospital) normally billed under Part B, which is described later in this chapter.

Medicare payments for covered services are made directly to the hospital and, except for the deductible and copayments, no further charge for covered services can be made to the beneficiary.

In October 1983, the basis for hospital reimbursement was changed from retrospective reimbursement of all costs to prospective payment on a fixed-price basis. Medicare pays hospitals a fixed amount for each patient stay based on the patient's admitting diagnosis. It uses 467 "diagnosis-related groups" (DRGs) to categorize these diagnoses. Each patient is assigned one DRG and the hospital receives a corresponding flat rate regardless of the number of days stayed or the services received. DRGs have reduced the length of time Medicare beneficiaries spend in the hospital and, because of this, charges of "premature discharge" have increased.

Private monitoring agencies called professional review organizations (PROs) play a major role in overseeing the hospital's treatment of Medicare patients. These PROs review the correctness of DRG information supplied by hospitals and the need for admission and extended care in certain cases. PROs also review hospital decisions that continuing an individual's care is no longer medically necessary.

If a Medicare beneficiary believes he or she is being prematurely discharged from a hospital, he or she should call the state's PRO office and request a review. A list of these PRO offices is available in *Your Medicare Handbook,* available free from your local Social Security office. The hospital may not bill the charges for the additional stay to the patient until the second day following the date of the discharge appeal, even if the review does not find the discharge in error.

Nursing home services. Medicare coverage for nursing home care has been severely restricted. Care in a skilled nursing facility (SNF) is covered only if all of the following conditions are met.

1. The patient has been hospitalized for at least 3 days in a row (within the 30-day period prior to nursing home admission).
2. The patient is transferred for further care for the condition that required hospitalization.
3. A doctor certifies the need for daily skilled nursing or rehabilitative services.
4. The SNF care is not disapproved by the facility's utilization review committee or the regional preadmission screening authority.

Once coverage is established, Medicare beneficiaries are eligible for up to 100 days of care in a skilled nursing facility per benefit period. But the average stay covered by Medicare is typically short. The beneficiary is required to make a copayment from the 20th day to the 100th day of Medicare-covered nursing home care. That copayment is $78.50 per day. As in the hospitalization benefit, the Medicare nursing home benefit covers most necessary items but no luxury items.

Home health services. Medicare does cover some home health care, with certain restrictions. One is that the beneficiary be homebound; another is that the services be on an intermittent, not a continuous, basis. It is no longer required that home health services follow a period of hospitalization. There is also no requirement that beneficiaries pay deductibles or copayments in connection with Medicare coverage of home health services.

Only "doctor-ordered" (necessary) medical services provided pursuant to a "plan of care" will be covered. Home health services must be provided by a licensed home health agency, which is Medicare-certified. Services covered include skilled nursing care and physical, occupational, and speech therapy. Home health aids may help the beneficiary with hygiene and nutrition. In addition some social services, medical equipment and supplies, and outpatient services can be covered by the home-health benefit.

This benefit does not cover home-delivered meals, full-time nursing care at home, medications, or homemaker services. The home-health benefit does not have deductibles or copayments. Patients must pay 20% of the approved cost for durable medical equipment, such as oxygen equipment, wheelchairs, and other equipment prescribed by a doctor.

Hospice services. Hospice care is designed for people who are terminally ill, with the goal of helping the patient and family deal with terminal illness. Part A covers hospice care for beneficiaries who are diagnosed as having a life expectancy of 6 months or less. Most services provided by a hospice are covered, including the services of staff doctors. To be eligible for hospice care, a beneficiary must elect to receive hospice care instead of most other Medicare benefits. Hospice benefits include nursing care, therapies, medical social services, medical supplies (including medication), respite care, and patient counseling.

For hospice care there is a 5% copayment for each respite care day and the lesser of a 5% or a $5 copayment for medication. Inpatient respite care is limited to 5 days in a row.

Part B: Medical Insurance

Medicare's medical insurance program for physician services is financed, in part, by monthly premiums paid by participants and in part by the federal government. The monthly premium in 1991 is $29.90. This premium is adjusted every January. There is also an annual deductible of $100 for the Part B benefit. There is also a charge for the first three unreplaced pints of blood used each year. Part B medical insurance pays 80% of Medicare-approved charges. In addition, Medicare beneficiaries are required to pay 20% copayments for most benefits, and whatever the physician or supplier charges over Medicare's "approved amount."

Medicare's approved amounts are fixed by the Health Care Financing Administration (HCFA). Many doctors prefer to charge higher rates than Medicare has approved. In this situation, the patient must pay the difference between the Medicare-approved charges and the physician's fees. The term "accepting assignment" is used to describe doctors who agree to set their fees at the Medicare-approved rates. If a physician does not ordinarily accept assignment, he or she may be willing to do so in a specific case if asked. Medicare provides a list of doctors and other health professionals who accept assignment for all Medicare beneficiaries. This is called the *Medicare Participating Physicians and Suppliers Directory.* It is available through the local Medicare intermediary in each state. These are listed in *Your Medicare Handbook.*

In addition to doctors' services, Medicare Part B covers a variety of other medical services. They include outpatient hospital services, emergency room services, rural health clinic services, outpatient rehabilitation, physical and occupational therapy, speech pathology services, prosthetic devices, and durable medical equipment, ambulance, X-ray treatment, and diagnostic tests, and some vaccinations. There is also coverage for the services of physician assistants and clinical psychologists who provide services through a community mental health center or a rural health clinic.

The Medicare program does not provide comprehensive coverage of the health care costs of the older adult. Besides the copayments and deductibles discussed earlier, Medicare specifically excludes some services that fall into the broad categories of routine or preventive care. These excluded services include most dental care, drugs (unless administered during covered treatment), routine physical examinations, eyeglasses and eyesight examinations, routine foot care, hearing exams, and most cosmetic surgery. Medicare also has a broad general exclusion and does not cover any service that is not "reasonable and necessary for the prevention of illness or injury." This can result in denial of coverage for services that beneficiaries might believe were covered.

The HCFA has an established appeals process for use by beneficiaries who believe a claim has been inappropriately denied. This process involves deadlines, and knowledgeable representation is advisable, so those who anticipate making an appeal should contact a legal service as soon as possible. For those 60 and over, the local AAA can identify the appropriate legal services office. A more complete description of the Medicare program can be found in *Your Medicare Handbook.*

Medicaid

Like Medicare, Medicaid was established under the 1965 amendments (Title XIX) to the Social Security Act. Unlike Medicare, Medicaid is a public assistance program with financial conditions of eligibility. The two programs also differ in their administration. Medicare is a federal program administered by an agency of the federal government. Direct administration of Medicaid, however, is carried out by each state. States vary in their eligibility requirements and in the medical services covered. Low-income older individuals may find it to their advantage to have both Medicare and Medicaid coverage.

Eligibility

Income and asset limits for Medicaid eligibility vary from state to state. Assets taken into account typically do not include a home, car, or personal property. Burial plots and money set aside for burial arrangements are also not treated as assets.

Given the high cost of nursing home care, families can quickly become impoverished after institutionalization of a loved one. To obtain Medicaid nursing home coverage, these families must *spend down* their monthly income and assets until they are eligible. This results in impoverishment of the remaining spouse (usually the wife). To address the problem of spousal impoverishment the Medicare Catastrophic Coverage Act (MCCA) of 1988 increased the amount of monthly income and assets that could be retained by a spouse. (The repeal of MCCA left this provision intact.) The amount of monthly income and assets the noninstitutionalized spouse may keep varies from state to state. As of 1990, the minimum amount states could permit the spouse to retain was a monthly allowance of $786. States may allow retention of as much as $1,565 monthly income. These amounts will increase to 150% of the federal poverty level for a couple in 1992.

The spouse also may retain at least $12,516 in assets. States, at their option, may allow up to $62,580 in assets to be retained. These amounts also will increase periodically. So, after the resources (not including home and personal property) are divided, those in excess of $12,516, or the asset limit set by the state if it is higher, are considered available to the institutionalized spouse. These "excess assets" must be spent before Medicaid will cover the cost of nursing home care.

Transfer of Assets

Some who anticipate needing Medicaid to cover nursing home care, but have too many assets, contemplate transferring their assets to their spouse or their children in order to become eligible. Just as it increased the resources available to the spouse of a nursing home patient, the MCCA of 1988 made laws regarding transfer of assets more stringent. Under this law, institutionalized patients are normally ineligible for Medicaid coverage if, within a period of 30 months prior to submitting an application for Medicaid, they disposed of resources for less than fair market value. This provision does not apply to a house transferred to a spouse, a child under 21 years of age, a disabled or blind adult child, an adult child who lived in the house and cared for the patient for at least 2 years before the patient was institutionalized, or a sibling who has equity in the house and lived in it for at least 1 year before nursing home placement.

If assets were transferred, Medicaid eligibility may be delayed by up to 30 months or the amount of time it would have taken to "spend down" the assets in question on nursing home care. Exceptions to these rules are made when a person can prove that reasonable attempts were made to obtain fair market value (to sell the asset) or the assets were not transferred to secure Medicaid coverage. Rules governing transfer of assets do not apply to money spent on needed services or goods.

Potential Medicaid applicants concerned with asset retention should seek legal advice from an attorney knowledgeable in Medicaid law. Many of these attorneys work in government-funded law offices and their services are free of charge (see the section on legal resources at the end of this chapter).

Eligibility for Medicaid can be retroactive. That is, states must pay for services provided to a Medicaid beneficiary during the 3 months prior to the month of application for Medicaid if the applicant was eligible for coverage during that period and requests retroactive payment on the application.

Services

Under federal law, states must provide Medicaid coverage for certain services and, at their option, may or may not provide for additional services under the Medicaid program. Mandatory services are:

inpatient hospital services,

outpatient hospital services and rural health clinic services,

laboratory and X-ray services,

skilled nursing facility services, and

physician services.

Optional services, which may (or may not) be covered by each state, include the following: home-health services, private duty nursing services, clinic services, dental services, physical therapy and related services, drugs, dentures, prosthetic devices, eyeglasses, diagnostic screening, preventive and rehabilitative services. In addition to these services, states are required to assure that transportation is available to those in need of medical care. A list of state Medicaid offices is presented at the end of this chapter.

Medigap Insurance

Medicare supplemental insurance policies (often called "Medigap" insurance) can be purchased to cover some expenses not entirely paid by Medicare. The coverage varies widely from policy to policy. Caregivers should know before purchase what expenses a policy does and does not cover.

Before purchasing a Medigap policy, caregivers must consider their financial resources and health. They may not need a supplemental policy if they are able to pay what Medicare does not. No one should purchase more than one Medicare supplement. Holding two or three policies is not normally cost-effective.

Typically, if Medicare does not cover a particular service, supplemental insurance will not either. Most Medigap insurance does not cover intermediate or custodial nursing home care, prescription drugs, eyeglasses, hearing aids, dentures, dental care, or routine physical examinations.

Medicare supplement policies generally only pay the unpaid portion (20%) of Medicare-approved charges. These are some questions to consider when comparing policies:

1. What are the pre-existing condition limitations, provisions, and waiting periods?
2. Does the policy cover physician charges above the Medicare-approved amount?
3. Does the policy pay Medicare Part A or B deductibles?

4. Is the policy "guaranteed renewable"? That is, can it be canceled if you get sick?

5. Will premiums increase each year?

6. Does the policy cover any medical services or supplies not covered by Medicare?

For more information on buying insurance to supplement Medicare, a pamphlet, "Guide to Health Insurance for People with Medicare," is available through the Consumer Information Center (listed in the resources section at the end of this chapter). Those who feel they have been victims of illegal sales practices should contact their state insurance department or call 1-800-638-6833 (in Maryland, 1-800-492-6603).

Long-Term Care Insurance

Several insurance companies offer long-term nursing care insurance policies to cover custodial (as opposed to rehabilitative) care in a nursing home. Custodial care is the level of care received by most nursing home residents. It involves help with the activities of daily living (ADL) such as eating, bathing, and dressing. Medicare does not pay for custodial care. Medicaid is the primary payer for custodial care for those unable to afford nursing home costs.

Long-term care insurance policies typically pay a fixed amount per day for nursing home care. Policies usually limit the number of days covered or restrict the total payment available.

Because the chances of using a nursing home increase with age, so do the premiums of long-term care insurance policies. Further, most policies currently offered have age limits. People over 79 years of age may not buy most policies. Most policies require a period of hospitalization prior to the nursing home stay, often a minimum of 3 days. Also, long-term care policies have an initial waiting period, usually 20 days, sometimes as long as 100 days. This means the policy does not pay its daily benefits for nursing home care during these initial waiting days.

Many policies do not cover mental diseases such as Alzheimer's, which are the most common cause of nursing home placement. Potential buyers should carefully consider the limitations of these policies and compare the costs and benefits in relation to obtaining Medicaid coverage for long-term care if necessary. For information on policies, insurance companies, or complaint resolution, contact your state insurance regulatory agency.

Legal Protective Arrangements

Several protective legal devices become relevant in situations of declining capacity. Some are voluntary and others are involuntary. Voluntary devices must be prepared by the person when he or she is competent. These include the living will and the durable power of attorney. The involuntary devices are imposed by courts for an individual who has lost capacity but did no prior planning. These court actions are generally of two types, guardianships and conservatorships.

Voluntary Actions

Living will. Many states recognize a living will or a "directive to physicians" as an appropriate way of controlling the nature of medical care a person will receive once he or she is in a terminal state *and* unable to communicate his or her wishes. A living will, unlike the traditional will described later in this chapter, does not affect the disposition of property.

Essentially, a living will is a document that provides directions to a patient's physician and family, helping to free them from the responsibility (and potential guilt) of making decisions about life-support equipment and medical procedures. Typically, the living will requests that "life-sustaining procedures" be withheld or withdrawn. It does not come into effect unless the patient is unable to communicate his or her desires.

Perhaps the most important aspect of a living will is the communication involved in preparing it. It is important that patients talk with their families and physicians about their wishes. Copies of the living will should be left with the spouse, doctor, and possibly with an attorney or executor for the family. Witnesses should not be relatives.

The living will also can specify a patient's wishes regarding organ donations. The Society for the Right to Die distributes a *Handbook of Living Will Laws,* which is periodically updated, and provides information on the laws in each state. The sources listed in the "Resources" section at the end of this chapter can help you obtain a living will.

Durable power of attorney. The durable power of attorney is used to give someone the legal authority to do something in the event that the person executing the document is unable. Powers of attorney may be time-limited or indefinite and the powers or authority they convey may be general or specific. One common use is to permit someone to cash income checks and pay bills on behalf of another. The durable power of attorney might be used to authorize a specific child to make important decisions regarding health care, or to handle some or all financial and legal affairs. To be binding, it must be notarized. Unlike simple powers of attorney, *durable* powers of attorney remain in effect when the person executing them becomes disabled or incompetent. The durable power of attorney is a fairly new legal device and may not be accepted in all states.

Involuntary Actions

Guardianship. Guardianship is an involuntary legal action initiated when an individual is not competent to care for him- or herself. A court appoints a guardian to be responsible for the well-being and/or the financial affairs of the ward (the incapacitated person). Sometimes separate guardians will be used, with one assuming responsibility for the person's well-being and another managing the finances. A guardianship proceeding is held in court; the person for whom guardianship is sought has a right to appeal. The guardian has a "fiduciary duty," meaning he or she is authorized only to act in the best interests of the ward.

A guardian can have the same relationship toward the ward as a parent has toward a young child. A guardian can have the authority to designate where the ward lives, what food he or she eats, what clothes he or she wears, and what medical care is appropriate.

Conservatorship. Conservatorship is like guardianship in that it involves a court procedure with the right to appeal. In conservatorship the court grants the conservator only the power to manage property, not the power to care for the personal affairs of the ward. Conservatorship procedures vary from state to state.

To preserve self-respect and individual rights, courts should grant only the powers that least restrict the ward's rights, yet are necessary to the ward's well-being. Conservatorships are an important way of preserving the ward's personal freedom while preventing waste or dissipation of assets through fraud or mismanagement.

Transferring Property

As people grow older, they are faced with planning for the distribution of property after their death. Some may want to give away property while they are still alive. Often, such transfers are motivated, in part, by the desire to have someone provide care during the later years.

If a person dies while owning real property (land and buildings) or a significant amount of other property, there probably will be a probate. A probate is a court proceeding that, among other things, transfers title to property from the person who has died to persons who survive. If there is a valid will, the property will be transferred according to the will. If there is no will, the property will be transferred according to state law. Probates can be slow and expensive. They are intended to ensure that the decedent's wishes are honestly and fully followed. But caregivers may wish to consider the alternatives to probate discussed below.

Sometimes taxes are due following a person's death. Under current law, federal taxes only apply if the "taxable estate" exceeds $600,000. The "taxable estate" is not limited to property owned at the time of death. It may include property the person once owned or had power over. For example, it might include gifts made "in contemplation of death" or property in which the decedent had retained an interest. Those who are close to the $600,000 limit should consult a lawyer. The modern trend is for states to impose death taxes only when the federal government does, but some states impose inheritance taxes even if inheritance is only a few thousand dollars.

Transferring property is more complicated than it may first appear. If possible, those involved should consult an attorney. Certain people (real estate agents, stockbrokers, and bank tellers, for example) may offer free advice. It is important to remember that their advice, though well intentioned, is generally accurate only as it relates to that person's area of expertise. It may ignore other, very important factors and therefore may be as bad as inaccurate advice.

Some ways to transfer property are described below.

Will. A will is a formal device for transferring property on death. It will usually require a probate. Wills generally must comply with technical rules to be valid. In other words, if a lawyer does not prepare a will, it may not be honored by the court if challenged.

A will can be changed at any time. In this respect, wills are more flexible than gifts, which, once made, are gone forever. The same formalities generally apply to changing wills as to making wills. If a will has been drawn up by an attorney, it is unwise to attempt to amend it without an attorney's assistance. Remember, a living will is not a will at all and is not a device to transfer property.

Trusts. Trusts are established by written instruments that involve three persons: (a) the person giving away the property (the grantor), (b) the person or legal entity who will take care of the property for a time (the trustee), and (c) the person or persons who will benefit from the gift (beneficiaries). A trust may be established in a will (a "testamentary trust") or by a written instrument executed during the grantor's life (a "living trust"). A living trust may be revocable (that is, you can change your mind later) or irrevocable. In a living trust, the grantor also may be the trustee. A revocable trust can avoid probate if the grantor is designated trustee, with a successor trustee designated to dispose of the property on the death of the grantor.

Some people avoid probate by lifetime gifts of property to their family. An outright gift is irrevocable. The giver has no legal right to take the property back, no matter what the other person does or does not do. A revocable trust may be a better idea. This can avoid probate, while allowing the giver to change his or her mind later.

A person may transfer property to a trust, serving as co-trustee with another person. If, in later years, the grantor becomes unable to manage the property, the co-trustee would manage it and pay for needed care without the necessity of court administration through a guardianship or conservator proceeding.

The trustee should always be someone trustworthy and known to the person. Caregivers may also choose to use an institutional trustee, such as a bank or a trust company, though there may be substantial fees for this.

Trusts can be set up so that after death, assistance can be given to a spouse, children, or grandchildren for living expenses, education, or otherwise, or even to provide gifts on birthdays, marriage, or other occasions. Trusts cannot go on forever, though, and it is often difficult to draft a trust for the benefit of a pet.

Joint tenancies. Property, usually real estate or securities, can be held by more than one person as "joint tenants with right of survivorship." On the death of one tenant, the survivor will be entitled to the property without probate when he or she can establish that the other tenant has died. This is a common way in which married couples hold property. (In community property states, such as California, it may be preferable for couples to hold assets as community property for tax reasons.)

A joint tenant can often force the sale of jointly held property if he or she decides to transfer his or her interest without the consent of the other joint tenant. Therefore, joint tenancies are not advisable unless there is an understanding about transfers and both tenants are willing to abide by it. Note also that creditors of either party may acquire an interest in the joint tenancy.

Bank accounts payable upon death (Totten trusts). Banks and other financial institutions generally offer accounts that give the depositor total control of the funds during life, but are payable (without probate) to a named survivor on the depositor's death. Those who open one of these accounts should be sure that the bank explains exactly how money can be withdrawn so that unauthorized withdrawals can be avoided.

Life estates. It is possible to transfer real property (such as a house) to someone else (for example, an adult child) retaining a "life estate." This means that the parent may live in the house during his or her life, but upon death the house will automatically belong to the child without probate.

This procedure involves executing and delivering a deed. Deeds, unlike wills, are generally irrevocable. That means if a parent deeds a house to a child, reserving a life estate, and later wants to leave the house to someone else (as for example, if the child does not provide good care to the parent), the parent cannot, because all the parent owns is the right to live in the home. A life estate may be a better idea than an absolute gift. With a life estate, the parent can use the home during his or her life. With an absolute gift, someone, including a creditor of the person who now owns the property, could force the parent to leave.

Contracts. Older people sometimes wish to strike a bargain with children, friends, or even total strangers. They might agree that certain property will go to the other person (again, perhaps a house) upon their death, provided the person takes care of them during their lifetime.

These arrangements are fraught with difficulty. For example, suppose a friend provides care for ten years and then has a falling out with the patient, who then wishes to leave the friend nothing. Will the patient be able to do this? Or, suppose, upon the patient's death, there is a contract (that is a document containing a promise) in which he or she agreed to leave the housekeeper the house in return for the care she has provided. Are the patient's children to believe that this is a genuine gift in appreciation of services rendered, or are they to think that the housekeeper took advantage of her position to deprive them of their inheritance? Or, suppose a person orally promises to leave a caregiver certain property, but dies, leaving nothing in writing. The property could very well go to people who had no part in the patient's care, leaving the person who did provide the care with nothing.

One way to handle these problems is to provide a fair reward now (e.g., salary) to the person providing care under a written contract stating that the salary is the only reward to which the person is entitled and that nothing will change this unless it is put in writing. A will can then be used if the patient wishes to add to the reward. The patient retains the option of changing the will.

Home Equity Conversions

Many older people and many caregivers are confronted with living on limited incomes while they have considerable home equity. Home equity conversion plans (HECs) are designed to provide cash for immediate use in exchange for equity in a home. These plans are new in the United States and are available only in a few areas. They may be either loan plans or sale plans.

Under loan plans, cash is made available, with payment due when a person moves out of the home or dies. Often loans are available for a specific purpose, such as making home repairs, remodeling, or paying property taxes. These special purpose loans are typically provided through public agencies, for those with limited incomes. In contrast, reverse mortgages, usually offered by private lenders, provide funds for any purpose, with no income restrictions. They usually are available at higher interest rates than are provided for special purpose loans.

Some HEC options involve selling the house with assurance that the older person will be permitted to live in it as long as he or she wishes.

HECs involve complicated legal and financial transactions, and should be approached with caution. When interest is compounded, a loan can quickly erode the equity in the home. Sometimes there is a risk that a long stay in a nursing home will trigger the repayment, which could force the older person to sell the home. Under some plans failure to properly maintain the home may result in eviction. Those contemplating an HEC will find an excellent review in a publication available through AARP entitled "Home-Made Money: Consumer's Guide to Home Equity Conversion."

This chapter is only an overview of some complicated and important laws and programs available. Caregivers should seek legal advice when necessary. Listed below are sources of free legal assistance. Private attorneys also practice in these areas of the law. The sources listed below can provide a referral to a private attorney if appropriate.

SUGGESTIONS FOR TRAINERS

In this session the following objectives apply:

1. Expose caregivers to legal devices including conservatorship, guardianship, durable power of attorney, living wills; and
2. Acquaint participants with sources of financial assistance such a Medicare, Medicaid, and private insurance.

I have found a guest speaker valuable in dealing with financial and legal issues. Leaders seldom have the training necessary to respond to individual questions that emerge during this presentation. A qualified speaker may come from several sources. A local AARP chapter may be able to provide a retired attorney who does volunteer work with older people. The State Office on Aging may have a staff person such as the nursing home ombudsman who regularly deals with these issues. The local bar association may have a speakers bureau. Finally, a legal service provider who works for an area agency on aging might give a presentation. Leaders should prepare the speaker to address issues specifically related to caregivers' situations. It is important that a guest speaker use minimal jargon and be sensitive to the lay person's anxiety regarding legal and financial issues.

STATE MEDICAID OFFICES

ALABAMA
Alabama Medicaid Agency
2500 Fairlane Drive
Montgomery, AL 36110
(205) 277-2710

ALASKA
Division of Medical Assistance
Department of Health and
Social Services
P.O. Box H
Juneau, AK 99811-0601
(907) 465-3030

ARIZONA
Arizona Health Care Cost
Containment System
(AHCCCS)
801 East Jefferson
Phoenix, AZ 85034
(602) 234-3655 ext. 4053

ARKANSAS
Office of Medical Services
Arkansas Dept. of Human
Services
P.O. Box 1437
Little Rock, AR 72203-1437
(501) 682-8292

CALIFORNIA
Medical Care Services
Department of Health Services
714 P Street, Room 1253
Sacramento, CA 95814
(916) 322-5824

COLORADO
Bureau of Medical Services
Department of Social Services
1575 Sherman, 6th Floor
Denver, CO 80203-1714
(303) 866-5901

CONNECTICUT
Medical Care Administration
Dept. of Income Maintenance
110 Bartholomew Avenue
Hartford, CT 06106
(203) 566-2934

DELAWARE
Dept. of Health and Social
Services
Delaware State Hospital
New Castle, DE 19720
(302) 421-6139

WASHINGTON, DC
Office of Health Care Financing
DC Dept. of Human Services
1331 H Street, N.W., Suite 500
Washington, DC 20005
(202) 727-0735

FLORIDA
Dept. of Health &
Rehabilitation Services
1317 Winewood Boulevard
Building 6, Room 233
Tallahassee, FL 32399-0700
(904) 488-3560

GEORGIA
Georgia Dept. of Medical
Assistance
2 Martin Luther King, Jr, Dr., SE
1220-C West Tower
Atlanta, GA 30334
(404) 656-4479

HAWAII
Health Care Administration
Division
Dept. of Human Services
P.O. Box 339
Honolulu, HI 96809
(808) 548-6584

IDAHO
   Bureau of Medical Assistance
   Dept. of Health and Welfare
   450 West State Street
   Statehouse Mail
   Boise, ID 83720
   (208) 334-5794

ILLINOIS
   Division of Medical Programs
   Illinois Dept. of Public Aid
   201 South Grand Avenue, East
   Springfield, IL 62743-0001
   (217) 782-2570

INDIANA
   Medicaid Division
   Indiana State Department
   of Public Welfare
   State Office Building, Room 702
   Indianapolis, IN 46204
   (317) 232-6865

IOWA
   Bureau of Medical Services
   Dept. of Human Services
   Hoover Street Office Bldg.,
   5th Floor
   Des Moines, IA 50319
   (515) 281-8694

KANSAS
   Medical Programs
   Dept. of Social and
   Rehabilitation Services
   Docking State Office Building
   Room 628-S
   Topeka, KS 66612
   (913) 296-3981

KENTUCKY
   Dept. of Medicaid Services
   3rd Floor
   275 East Main Street
   Frankfort, KY 40621
   (502) 564-4321

LOUISIANA
   Bureau of Health Services
   Financing
   P.O. Box 91030
   Baton Rouge, LA 70821-9030
   (504) 342-3891

MAINE
   Bureau of Medical Services
   Dept. of Human Services
   State House, Station 11
   Augusta, ME 04333
   (207) 289-2674

MARYLAND
   Health Care Policy, Financing
   and Regulation
   Dept. of Health and
   Mental Hygiene
   201 West Preston Street,
   Room 525
   Baltimore, MD 21201
   (301) 225-6535

MASSACHUSETTS
   Department of Public Welfare
   180 Tremont Street, 13th Floor
   Boston, MA 02111
   (617) 574-0202

MICHIGAN
   Medical Services Administration
   Dept. of Social Services
   P.O. Box 30037
   Lansing, MI 48909
   (517) 335-5001

MINNESOTA
   Health Care Programs Division
   Department of Human Services
   444 Lafayette Road, 6th Floor
   St. Paul, MN 55155-3848
   (612) 296-2766

MISSISSIPPI
Division of Medicaid
Office of the Governor
801 Robert E. Lee Building
239 North Lamar Street
Jackson, MS 39201-1311
(601) 359-6050

MISSOURI
Division of Medical Services
Dept. of Social Services
P.O. Box 6500
Jefferson City, MO 65102
(314) 751-6529

MONTANA
Medical Services Division
Dept. of Social and
Rehabilitation Services
P.O. Box 4210
Helena, MT 59604
(406) 444-4540

NEBRASKA
Medical Services Division
Dept. of Social Services
5th Floor
301 Centennial Mall South
Lincoln, NE 68509
(402) 471-9330

NEW HAMPSHIRE
Office of Medical Services
New Hampshire Division of
Human Services
Dept. of Health and Human Services
6 Hazen Drive
Concord, NH 03301-6521
(603) 271-4353

NEW JERSEY
Division of Medical Assistance
and Health Services
Department of Human Services
CN-712, 7 Quakerbridge Plaza
Trenton, NJ 08625
(609) 588-2602

NEW MEXICO
Medical Assistance Division
Human Services Department
P.O. Box 2348
Santa Fe, NM 87504-2348
(505) 827-4315

NEW YORK
Division of Medical Assistance
New York State Department
of Social Services
Ten Eyck Office Building
40 North Pearl Street
Albany, NY 12243-0001
(518) 474-9132

NORTH CAROLINA
Division of Medical Assistance
Department of Human Resources
1985 Umstead Drive
Raleigh, NC 27603
(919) 733-2060

NORTH DAKOTA
Medical Services
North Dakota Department of
Human Services
600 East Boulevard
Bismarck, ND 58505-0261
(701) 224-2321

OHIO
Benefits Administration
Medicaid Administration
Dept. of Human Services
30 East Broad Street, 31st Floor
Columbus, OH 43266-0423
(614) 466-3196

OKLAHOMA
Division of Medical Services
Dept. of Human Services
P.O. Box 25352
Oklahoma City, OK 73125
(405) 557-2539

OREGON
Senior and Disabled Services
Division
Dept. of Human Resources
313 Public Service Building
Salem, OR 97310
(503) 378-4728

PENNSYLVANIA
Medical Assistance Programs
Room 515
Dept. of Public Welfare
Health and Welfare Building
Harrisburg, PA 17105-2675
(717) 787-1870

RHODE ISLAND
Division of Medical Services
Department of Human Services
600 New London Avenue
Cranston, RI 02920
(401) 464-3575

SOUTH CAROLINA
South Carolina State Health and
Human Services
Finance Commission
P.O. Box 8206
Columbia, SC 29202-8206
(803) 253-6100

SOUTH DAKOTA
Medical Services
Dept. of Social Services
Kneip Building
700 Governors Drive
Pierre, SD 57501-2291
(605) 773-3495

TENNESSEE
Bureau of Medicaid
729 Church Street
Nashville, TN 37219
(615) 741-0213

TEXAS
Dept. of Human Services
P.O. Box 149030
Austin, TX 78714-9030
(512) 450-3050

UTAH
Div. of Health Care Financing
Utah Department of Health
P.O. Box 16580
Salt Lake City, UT 84116-0580
(801) 538-6151

VERMONT
Dept. of Social Welfare
Vermont Agency of Human
Services
103 South Main Street
Waterbury, VT 05676
(802) 241-2880

VIRGINIA
Virginia Dept. of Medical
Assistance Services
600 East Broad Street
Suite 1300
Richmond, VA 23219
(804) 786-7933

VIRGIN ISLANDS
Bureau of Health Insurance
and Medical Assistance
Knud Hansen Complex
Charlotte Amalie
St. Thomas, VI 00802
(809) 774-4624

WASHINGTON
Division of Medical Assistance
Dept. of Social & Health Services
623 8th Avenue, S.E.
Mail Stop HB-41
Olympia, WA 89504
(206) 753-1777

WEST VIRGINIA
  Division of Medical Care
  West Virginia Dept. of
  Human Services
  1900 Washington Street, East
  Charleston, WV 25305
  (304) 348-8990

WISCONSIN
  Bureau of Health Care Financing
  Division of Health
  Wisconsin Dept. of Health
  and Social Services
  P.O. Box 309
  Madison, WI 53701-0309
  (608) 266-2522

WYOMING
  Medical Assistance Services
  Dept. of Health and
  Social Services
  Hathaway Building, 4th Floor
  Cheyenne, WY 82002-0710
  (307) 777-7531

RESOURCES

Books

Your Medicare Handbook. A wonderful place to start if you have questions about Medicare. Available through the local Social Security office.

Matthews, J. L., & Matthews, D. B. (1990). *Social Security, Medicare and pensions,* (5th ed.). Berkeley, CA: Nolo Press. (800) 992-NOLO.

Waller, K. (1981). *How to recover your medical expenses: A comprehensive guide to understanding and unscrambling Medicare.* New York: Collier Books.

Organizations

  Consumer Information Center
  Department 59
  Pueblo, CO 81009

For publications about Medicare and Health Insurance for people with Medicare.

American Association for Retired Persons (AARP)
1909 K Street, N.W.
Washington, DC 20049

Society for the Right to Die
250 West 57 Street
New York, NY 10107

Contact this organization for the *Handbook of Living Will Laws.*

Sources of Legal Assistance

Aging agencies. Area Agencies on Aging fund legal assistance for civil matters, such as public benefits representation, consumer issues, and medical help. AAA lawyers provide limited assistance to citizens 60 and older, of any income level. To locate such legal aid, call a local senior citizens center or aging services office, usually listed in the county or city section of the phone directory.

Legal Services Corporations. Each state has a local Legal Services office, which provides free civil legal representation (not criminal) in limited areas of the law. Certain services are available to low-income individuals of all ages, and older people of all incomes. The aging services office can refer you to the local Legal Services office.

County Attorney. County Attorneys are employed to handle matters mandated to counties by law. For example, County Attorneys may be responsible for initiating guardianship and conservatorship actions for those lacking parties to act in their interest. County Attorneys are also excellent sources of referral for all types of legal problems. Their phone numbers will be listed in the phone directory under county government offices.

Chapter 8

CAREGIVING SKILLS

Many caregivers appreciate and benefit from learning specific skills. Those who are reluctant to participate in a program designed to reduce their stress will often sign up to learn to do a better job of care- giving. This seems especially true of men. This chapter addresses two areas: medication management and home safety. It does not address techniques for personal care, such as transferring or bathing a patient. These are best learned individually from a health care provider, as they will vary a great deal according to the physical condition of both caregiver and care receiver.

MEDICATION MANAGEMENT

To manage effectively both their own and the care receiver's medications, caregivers need to have a basic knowledge of prescription and over-the-counter drugs, as well as guidelines for discussing medications with their physician. This section provides general information about side effects, drug interactions, misuse of drugs, generic drugs, and over-the-counter medications. Tables 8.1 and 8.2 address the "dos and don'ts" of prescription and over-the-counter drugs.

A drug is any chemical that alters the way the body works. A medicine is a drug or a combination of drugs that is used for medical purposes. Medicines do not cure diseases; they may help the body control a disease (for example: antibiotics help fight infection), they may reduce the symptoms of a disease (aspirin reduces pain), or they may be used to prevent certain conditions (Warfarin, also called *Coumadin*, prevents blood clots).

Drugs are powerful substances, with the capacity for great help and great harm. There is no known drug that is not harmful or toxic at high doses. So, all drugs are poisons. The words "poison" and "potion" come from the Greek word *pharmakon*, which means a substance that could either heal or hurt.

Side Effects

Every drug can cause unintended effects. Side effects are usually unwanted and unpleasant, such as dry mouth, blurred vision, drowsiness, and nausea. Some may be insidious, like loss of appetite, confusion, and depression. Side effects often occur shortly after a person starts taking a drug, but they can appear after an extended period of use. Caregivers need to be especially alert for side effects that appear long after the patient has begun using a drug. Usually these delayed side effects are the most difficult to pinpoint. Caregivers must be careful to avoid attributing confusion or depression to illness or advanced age. It is always worthwhile to ask the physician or pharmacist whether such changes might be caused by a medication.

It is important to discuss possible side effects prior to taking the medication. The caregiver should be assured that the potential benefits of the drug outweigh its potential side effects. The caregiver also needs to be aware of what to expect and what to do in the event of side effects.

Drug Interactions

Multiple drug use greatly increases the likelihood of drug interactions and drug misuse. Upon discharge from a hospital, 25% of older patients receive prescriptions for six or more drugs, and it is not uncommon to find some older patients using 12 to 15 prescription drugs (Sloan, 1986). It can be difficult to keep track of the schedule for taking a variety of pills, which increases the likelihood of failing to comply with instructions. Further, the elderly often receive prescriptions from several specialists, and it is rare that any single health provider keeps track of the various drugs prescribed by the others. This places the patient at risk of drug interactions. As a result, the

ery drugs that are supposed to make a person well can prove un-
ealthy, even lethal.

Drugs can interact with every other thing we put into our bodies.
'hey can interact with other drugs, either increasing or decreasing
heir effect. They can interact with food. Usually if a drug is taken
vith food absorption is slowed. This means it takes longer for the
lrug to take effect. Drugs often interact with alcohol. Usually alcohol
ncreases the drug's impact. This not only applies to the alcohol in
lrinks, but also to the alcohol in cold preparations. Drugs also can
nteract with tobacco.

Misuse of Drugs

Misuse refers to any activity that is not consistent with the intended
ise of the drug. Many hospital admissions are the direct result of
misuse of drugs. In a recent study about 10% of older patients admitted to hospitals were suffering from adverse drug reactions (Sloan,
1986). Many common practices constitute misuse: under- or over-
ising a prescribed drug, sharing medications with a friend, saving
medications beyond their expiration date, stopping abruptly without
consulting a physician, and failing to comply with directions for taking a medicine.

Over- or under-use of a prescribed drug. It is complicated to determine
the appropriate dose for use by an older person. This is because physiological changes that come with age affect the absorption, distribution,
metabolism, and excretion of drugs. Older people sometimes absorb drugs
at a lower rate. This means it takes longer before the drug's effect is felt.
Either patient or caregiver may become impatient or worried, waiting for
the drug to "kick in," and decide to take some more. This over-use and
the slower metabolism may create a "hangover effect," with the drug
staying in the body much longer than intended. Both caregiver and care
receiver need to be aware of how long they will need to wait before the
drug takes effect.

Under-use is often done to save money. An older patient may find
the symptoms diminishing and decide to save money by cutting back
on the dosage. But, with antibiotics, for example, symptoms may
abate before an infection is completely eradicated. Discontinuing the
medication may lead to relapse. When money is a concern, it is
worthwhile to discuss cost-effective alternatives with both the prescribing physician and the pharmacist.

Sharing medications with a friend. Again, in efforts to economize, peopl may exchange medications with friends who have similar symptoms. This i problematic for several reasons. First, similar symptoms may not have th same cause; second, dosage may be inappropriate; and finally, the medicatio may have expired.

Saving medications. Most medicine cabinets in America have at least on expired drug. In part this is because we are reluctant to throw away anythin, that works, and in part because we cannot imagine a drug "expiring." Drug like food, "spoil." Their chemical composition changes and they becom ineffective or even dangerous. This is particularly true when drugs ar stored in a humid place, such as the bathroom cabinet, or in sunlight, suc as the kitchen window sill.

Discontinuing abruptly. People sometimes discontinue a drug abruptl because they no longer experience the symptoms that led them to take th drug, they run out and are unable to refill the prescription, or they experienc unpleasant side effects. Yet abruptly stopping some medications is ex tremely dangerous. For example, anti-anxiety agents can cause con vulsions if discontinued suddenly. If a refill is prescribed, caregiver should get the refill well before running out of the initial prescription.

Failing to comply with directions. A major reason for noncompliance i that the person taking the drug never understood the directions. Pharmacist estimate that as many as 50% of patients do not know how to take the dru when the prescription for it is filled.

Other reasons for noncompliance relate to sensory loss, confusion. and functional problems such as arthritis. It can be very difficult tc read the small print on medicine containers. Arthritis can make i nearly impossible to open safety caps. And, when a person is taking several medications it takes only a little confusion to make a mistake.

Caregivers can reduce the chance of noncompliance in three ways:

1. Be sure the care receiver understands how a medication should be taken.

2. Work with the physician to develop a medication regime the care receiver can live with. This may involve requesting non-safety caps if children are not in the house, asking for medication that does not have to be given as often, or asking if a medication is available in a more manageable form (for example, liquid preparations may be available for a patient who has difficulty swallow-ing pills). Caregivers who have difficulty complying with the doctor's orders should ask the doctor whether the orders can be changed.

3. Use mnemonic devices to ensure proper dosage. Many pharmacists can suggest ways to keep track of medications. These might involve developing

a drug reminder calendar, or organizing the day's or week's pills in a container such as an egg carton or a dated pill box (see Table 8.1).

Over-the-Counter Drugs

Watch TV for a few minutes and you learn how to spell "relief." Over-the-counter medications are available to anyone without the supervision of a physician (prescription). There are currently 350,000 over-the-counter drugs on the market, but these products only contain about 500 different "active ingredients" (medicines). The media encourages us to believe that all over-the-counter drugs are safe and effective. While often true, the Food and Drug Administration, in an extensive review of over-the-counter preparations, found only 30% to 40% were safe and effective for the problem they were designed to address.

Misuse, or inappropriate use of these drugs, is dangerous. They should be used only for the relief of minor and *temporary* symptoms. Used for this purpose, their advantages are that they are relatively inexpensive, convenient, and may even provide relief. The disadvantages are the possibility of drug interactions, side effects, and masking symptoms of a serious illness (see Table 8.2).

Generic Drugs

Many drugs are available under two names—the trade name and the generic name. The trade name refers to the brand name of the medication or the name of the manufacturer. The generic name refers to the drug compound itself, without regard to the brand name. Today in the United States all rights to market a new drug may be protected for 22 years following issue of a patent. During this period, the originating firm has exclusive rights to produce the drug. After the patent has expired any manufacturer may market the drug using its generic name.

Generic drugs should be used with caution. Approved generics sometimes have potencies that differ from the trade drug. Because of this possibility patients who use generics should stick with the same generic. Generic drugs are not all as effective as trade drugs, and some are not less expensive. It is important to ask both a physician and a pharmacist before substituting a generic drug.

Table 8.1
Dos and Don'ts of Prescription Drug Use

Do:

1. *Keep a list of medications,* including over-the-counter medicines. This is useful to share with physicians and will help reduce the risk of drug interactions.

2. *Understand directions* before leaving the physician's office. This includes knowing whether a generic might be used, how to take the medication (does three times a day mean every 8 hours in a 24-hour period or three times during waking hours?); what side effects might occur; what to do about side effects; and what to do if a dose is missed.

3. *Ask about driving, food, and alcohol.* Can you drive while using this medication? Does it require a full or empty stomach? Will it interact with alcohol?

4. *Take all medications with a full glass of water.* Some drugs (like aspirin) can damage the esophagus if they remain in contact. Also, the liquid helps the medication dissolve in the stomach.

5. *Report any side effects to the prescribing physician* (this includes insidious effects that may or may not be due to the drug).

6. *Minimize the number of different drugs used.* This will reduce the risk of interactions. A regular medication review should be conducted to determine if a drug is still needed.

7. *Take medicine bottles when visiting the physician* (this includes over-the-counter medicines as well as vitamins).

8. *Ask questions.* It does not hurt to ask the pharmacist the same questions you asked the physician. Pharmacists may have a different perspective, or more recent information about the drug.

9. *Report any compliance problems to the physician.* This includes a tendency to forget the medicine, as well as difficulty with the dosage form (pills versus liquids).

10. *Discard medicines when they expire.* They spoil just like food.

Don't:

1. *Don't share medicine with friends.* Friends have different ailments and bodies. Share good times, instead.

2. *Don't store medicine in the bathroom.* It is too humid, and often close to the bedroom. This means midnight doses may be taken without waking up — with resulting mistakes. Store medicine in the kitchen, or someplace at a distance from the bedroom.

3. *Don't take medicine in the dark.* Use a magnifying glass to read the label, if necessary.

Table 8.2
Dos and Don'ts for Over-the-Counter Medications

Do:

1. Ask a physician or pharmacist whether the medication is the right one for you, particularly if buying a cold or cough preparation. Many of these contain multiple ingredients that could be dangerous.
2. Read the label every time you purchase a medication.
3. Treat over-the-counter preparations with the same caution that applies to prescription drugs. Follow directions carefully, and be alert for side effects.
4. Use over-the-counter medicine only for minor and temporary symptoms.

Don't:

1. Don't use any over-the-counter drug for more than one week unless advised by a physician.
2. Don't believe all the advertising claims made by manufacturers.
3. Don't drive or use alcohol when taking tranquilizers, sedatives, antihistamines, or pain medication. They can make you drowsy.

HOME SAFETY

Caregivers can accommodate some physical limitations experienced by patients by modifying the home environment. These home safety measures will reduce the likelihood of accidents and enhance the independence of care receivers.

Lighting

Because of changes in the eye, most older people are less able to adjust to changes in lighting and are more sensitive to glare. Night vision is often impaired. Visual changes also can reduce sensitivity to contrasts. This means that light-colored objects on light-colored floors become invisible, and the subtle difference between the end of one stair and the beginning of the next can go undetected.

Several steps can be taken to accommodate these changes.

1. Reduce glare. This can be done by minimizing the number of shiny surfaces (furniture tops and floors). Shiny surfaces can be waxed with nonglare finishes,

or shiny furniture can be moved away from light sources. Glare from outside light can be reduced without losing a view of the outdoors through use of sheer curtains.

2. Install night-lights. These are particularly important in bedroom, bathroom, and kitchen areas.
3. Intensify contrasts. For example, strips of contrasting tape can be installed at the edges of steps to make them more visible.

Mobility

When an older person suffers from mobility limitations it is important to reduce the likelihood of tripping. Objects left on the floor, such as reading material, clothing, or tools, need to be kept on tables or shelves. Electric cords should be removed from trafficked areas. Throw rugs should be eliminated or taped to the floor so they don't slide. Stairs should be kept free of clutter. Overstuffed and low furniture can entrap an older person, reducing opportunities for mobility. Sharp corners on furniture can be padded or moved from heavily trafficked areas.

Bathroom Safety

The combination of water and slick surfaces in most bathrooms can be a major hazard. Adaptive devices can be installed to prevent falls. These include a rubber mat on the shower floor or in front of the toilet; a hydraulic tub chair to lower the patient into the bath; rails in the tub and near the toilet to make it easier to get up; and raised toilet seats. Lowering the thermostat on the hot water heater minimizes the risk of scalding.

Kitchen Safety

The kitchen has many potential hazards, including things that can cut or burn a person. The stove can be adapted through installation of a cutoff switch that prevents unsupervised use, or the burner control handles can be removed. For the visually impaired, dials can be marked with red tape or paint placed in the cooking position most often used. Condiments that are often used can be relabeled with large print or put in special containers to prevent mistakes. When cooking, handles of pots and pans should not stick out from the edge. Someone passing by could brush against a handle, burning him- or herself. Cleaning agents, such as automatic dishwashing detergent, should be put away, and nonfood items kept separate from food items.

Safety for the Cognitively Impaired

The unique problems confronted by those who care for the cognitively impaired are thoroughly addressed in a book by Mace and Rabins, *The 36-Hour Day* (1981). They present suggestions for managing these problems and creating a safe home environment. Here are some examples.

1. Install devices that make it difficult to open outside doors, such as hooks at the top of the door or plastic door knobs that must be squeezed to open the door
2. Install bells on doors so caregivers will be aware when they are opened
3. Unplug major appliances, such as the stove and oven
4. Use labels and pictures to remind patients of the use of objects, such as the toilet or refrigerator

A note on smoking. Unsupervised smoking can represent a significant hazard. This is true, not just of cognitively impaired elderly, but of anyone who might forget that a cigarette is lit or fall asleep while smoking. Caregivers can minimize this hazard by removing cigarettes and matches when they cannot supervise their use.

Gadgets

An incredible array of gadgets, many homemade, can be used to make life easier and safer for the disabled. Some of these are elaborate, such as a tip-up chair, which has springs that raise it up when weight is leaned forward. Others are simple. Simple aids include the following:

- Wrist straps that can be taped onto canes to make them easier to retrieve
- A kitchen chair trolley, made of an upright chair with castors—the chair gives some support, and articles can be carried on the seat
- An apron with pockets, which can be used to carry objects around the home
- A wide range of dishes and cutlery, including plate rims, silverware with enlarged handles, and "no-grip" cutlery that attaches to the hand with velcro
- A suction cup, which can be applied to the bottom of dishes to prevent slipping
- Toilet tongs, a pair of kitchen tongs that can be used to hold toilet paper or other cleansing material, and makes reaching easier

The number of manufactured devices has grown considerably in recent years. Caregivers should refer to the Sears Home Health Catalogue (available by calling 1-800-366-3000) and medical supply stores in their area to learn about the latest aids on the market.

SUGGESTIONS FOR TRAINERS

A session on caregiver skills can address the following objectives:

1. Improve participants' skill in medication management and home safety
2. Satisfy participants' desire to justify training on the basis of care recipients' needs
3. Support caregivers' sense of efficacy by acknowledging they're already doing a good job

Many caregivers will enroll in a training program only to improve their skills, so this session will encourage participation. It is deliberately placed late in the training program to maintain attendance. New information about how to "do" caregiving may arouse guilt, even resentment. Participants may respond to the content as an implicit criticism of the way they have been doing things. This can be defused by acknowledging soon that they may be doing things differently, and they may or may not choose to adopt the new skills being presented.

Because medication management is such an important skill, a guest speaker may be helpful in this area. A pharmacist can provide the presentation, then provide a medication review for participants. Participants should bring everything in their medicine cabinet (both over-the-counter and prescription medications) to the session in a paper bag. Then, while small groups are practicing a communication skill, individuals meet with the pharmacists for a review of their medications. The pharmacist can identify potential drug interaction problems and counsel caregivers about failure to comply with doctors' orders.

RESOURCES

La Buda, Dennis R. (Ed.). (1985). *The gadget book: Ingenious devices for easier living.* Washington, DC: American Association of Retired Persons.

Medication Management

Smith, Dorothy, L. (1987). *Understanding prescription drugs*. New York: Pocket Books.

Home Safety

"Coping and Home Safety Tips for Caregivers of the Elderly." A video with accompanying manual available through

Jefferson Area Board for Aging
423 Lexington Avenue
Charlottesville, VA 22901
(804) 978-3644

"Home Safety checklist for older consumers" (1985). U.S. Department of Health and Human Services and U.S. Consumer Product Safety Commission, Washington, DC.

For the Cognitively Impaired

Mace, N. L., & Rabins, P. V. (1981). *The 36-hour day: A family guide to caring for persons with Alzheimer's disease, related dementing illnesses, and memory loss in later life.* Baltimore, MD: Johns Hopkins University Press.

Chapter 9

GRIEF AND DYING

And ever it has been that love knows not its own depth until the hour of separation.

Kahlil Gibran, *The Prophet*

Grieving is an important yet often neglected task of caregiving. Both caregivers and care receivers experience losses ranging from immediate, physical loss to anticipated, symbolic loss. It is important to grieve these losses. By giving themselves and their loved ones permission to grieve, caregivers improve the quality of their relationships and their lives. Further, caregivers can prepare for the death of a loved one by learning what they might expect of themselves during bereavement.

The term "anticipatory grief" has been used to describe the grief experienced by those caring for terminally ill patients as well as by the patients themselves. This term is controversial and, several authors have argued, a contradiction in terms (see Parkes & Weiss, 1983; Silverman, 1974). How, after all, can we grieve over a loss that we have not yet experienced? Caregivers themselves may wonder why they experience a sense of loss when they have not yet faced the death of their loved one.

The grief experienced by caregivers is only partially "anticipatory," referring to a future as opposed to a present loss. Because the death of the care receiver overshadows other losses, caregivers may not grieve the very real losses they have experienced. Yet by allowing themselves to grieve these losses, caregivers can to some extent prepare themselves for the death of their loved ones.

E. M. Pattison (1977) described the experience of dying by referring to the three phases diagrammed in Figure 9.1. Following an initial period of acute crisis, the family enters into what Pattison called the "living-dying" phase. The final, "terminal" phase of the process immediately precedes the time of death. This approach is useful for organizing our discussions; but dying, like living, seldom follows such a tidy trajectory. Although his work focused on the reaction of the patient, the three phases also can be used to describe the experiences of family members and friends. Therese Rando pointed out, "When a loved one is dying, so too are the other family members" (1986, p. 97). Family members are likely to move back and forth among three phases Pattison described, sometimes experiencing more than one at the same time.

DIAGNOSIS AND THE PHASE
OF ACUTE CRISIS

The diagnosis of a life-threatening disease often presents an acute crisis, with accompanying feelings of shock, numbness, and disbelief. (I use the term "disbelief" instead of the more common term "denial." This is because denial frequently assumes value-laden and negative connotations. It implies the person deliberately ignores reality and must be helped to face it. Disbelief is a gentler term, emphasizing the difficulty we have coming to grips with threatening information.) Sometimes this disbelief translates into a search for the right test or the right doctor—that is, one who can tell the family that this is not really happening. Although health professionals may be inclined to dismiss this search as an irrational waste of time, money, and energy, it does serve two important purposes. First, it provides an opportunity to review and confirm the diagnosis. This is particularly important with diseases such as Alzheimer's, which can be misdiagnosed. Second, it provides a buffer—postponing the time when the family must face and begin to cope with the harsh reality confronting them.

Hope emerges as a central theme for those who confront death. Without it, the process of loss is truly unbearable. During this acute crisis period, the hope is that either the diagnosis or the prognosis is

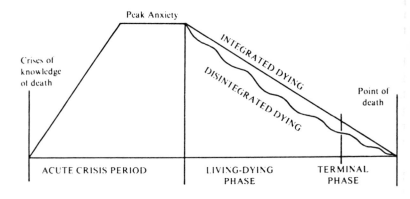

Figure 9.1. The Experience of Dying
SOURCE: E. M. Pattison. *The Experience of Dying* (p. 44). Englewood Cliffs, NJ: Prentice-Hall.

incorrect. "This isn't really Alzheimer's," or "I may have leukemia, but it won't kill me. I'll beat the odds." Later, the hope for a better prognosis receives periodic boosts if the patient seems to be doing especially well or experiences a remission. The surges of hope become an emotional roller coaster that will become familiar to all involved. Ultimately, the content of hope may shift to acknowledge the reality of dying. Patients and family members may then hope that death will wait until certain significant events have passed, or that the death will be dignified, appropriate, and as painless as possible.

Whenever possible, major decisions should be postponed during a phase of acute crisis. It is difficult, if not impossible, for family members to concentrate on complex information about treatment and care options when they are experiencing a whirlwind of emotions.

THE "LIVING-DYING" PHASE

Most caregiving takes place during the second, "living-dying" phase of dying. During this time caregivers and care receivers need permission and support to grieve the losses they are experiencing. Admittedly they have not yet confronted death, but they have lost life as they once knew it.

Caregivers have lost a healthy family member, who could have been their source of strength and companionship. They have lost the freedom to take time for granted. They have lost control, not just of the future but of their daily lives. They have lost their dreams of the future they planned to share with their loved one. They may have already lost some of their roles, such as the role of wife of a successful working man.

Care receivers experience similar losses, accompanied by the expectation that they will be losing everything. Their lives and those of their families have been taken over by a disease. During this time the everyday routine is punctuated by visits to the physician, schedules for treatment and medication, and concerns about their side effects.

Ambivalence

This period is marked by ambivalent emotions that have their roots in the profound dilemmas caregivers encounter. Support for grieving caregivers requires acknowledging the dilemmas they face. Therese Rando (1986, pp. 101-102) described some of these:

> Increasing attachment to the patient during the illness vs. starting to decathect from the patient in terms of his or her existence in the future; . . . planning for life after the death of the patient vs. not wanting to betray the patient by considering life in his or her absence; communicating feelings to the patient vs. not wanting to make the patient feel guilty for dying or bound to this world when the patient needs to let go; . . . focusing on the past and recollecting with the patient vs. focusing on the future; . . . redistributing family roles and responsibilities vs. not wanting to do anything that would call attention to or cause more losses for the patient; . . . being immersed in participating in the patient's care vs. living one's own life; . . . identifying a loss so it can be grieved by the patient vs. focusing more positively on the remaining potentials.

Central to these dilemmas is the perceived conflict between the need to reorganize and survive the death of the loved one and the desire to provide loving, hopeful care. These dilemmas emerge because we tend to see the two tasks as incompatible. We may see our suffering as proof of our love or as punishment for our failings (see the "Guilt" section in this chapter). With this understanding in mind, we can more readily cope with these dilemmas. This is facilitated when the "versus" is replaced by "and." For example: Caregivers can expect to feel increasing attachment to the patient during the illness *and* it is important that they begin to "decathect" (disengage) from the patient in terms of future expectations. Caregivers need to be immersed in the patient's care *and* they need to live their own lives. The caregiver's task is not one of choosing between two opposing values, but one of balancing needs and allocating resources.

Anger and Resentment

Anger is a natural reaction to loss. Yet many of us have been taught that anger is not socially acceptable and, as a result, we do not know how to use our anger constructively. Our first reaction may be to want to stop feeling anger. We may deny it exists or turn it upon ourselves in episodes of brutal self-criticism. A training program can legitimize caregivers' angry feelings and support appropriate expression. Leo Madow said, "Anger is an energy. It cannot be destroyed or forgotten. It has to be converted" (Stearns, 1984, p. 59). Anger can be channeled in constructive ways. For example, caregivers might be encouraged to use exercise as an outlet for their emotions, or they might be encouraged to use it to energize their advocacy efforts.

Caregivers may become angry with the person who is ill and feel abandoned or betrayed by the patient. About a third of the participants in CSP reported feeling resentful of their spouses. Most did not know how to cope with such feelings. Many tried to talk themselves out of their feelings by reminding themselves that "his (or her) problems are worse than mine." Those who could not talk themselves out of it just lived with their feelings of anger and resentment. Some found physical activity an effective outlet.

Caregivers also may become angry with the God they believe let (or made) this happen to them and their loved ones. This anger can be especially difficult for those who have previously found strength and consolation in their faith. Rather than question the unfairness or cruelty of God, some caregivers may search their histories for the personal failing that made them "deserve" such cruel treatment, or they may blame the patient for bringing it on himself or herself. In these circumstances, anger creates a crisis of faith. Rabbi Kushner's book *When Bad Things Happen to Good People* (1981) provides a useful perspective for coping with this type of crisis.

When caregivers become angry with professionals, the professionals tend to assume this is "displaced anger." That is, because it is socially or personally unacceptable to be angry with the patient or with God, caregivers take it out on their doctors or social workers. Sometimes this may be true. But it is important to acknowledge that caregivers may be justifiably angry with professionals who fail to meet their needs for support and care.

Guilt

It is ironic that caregivers, who work a 36-hour day, frequently experience guilt. There are three sources of this guilt. Most who feel guilty believe that their caregiving is inadequate. They would like to be able to do more for their loved one, although in some cases they are already exceeding their physical abilities. Some are motivated to participate in training because of the guilt that they feel about their supposedly inadequate caregiving. Another source of guilt is negative feelings toward the patient. Caregivers who resent the patient's dependency or illness frequently feel guilty about that resentment. Still other caregivers feel responsible for their loved one's illness. This is reminiscent of the "magical thinking" that presents problems for bereaved children who have wished that their parents would die. It takes a more concrete form in adults. One of the CSP participants illustrated this when she said, "If only I hadn't cooked such rich foods . . . he would never have gotten sick."

Guilt can seriously complicate grieving after the death of the loved one. In a sense, the period of anticipatory grief provides an opportunity to address guilt as well as other "unfinished business." It is difficult to talk people out of their feelings of guilt. Better to help them forgive themselves. For specific approaches to forgiveness, see *Guilt: Letting Go,* by Lucy Freeman and Herbert Strean (1986), listed in the resource section at the end of this chapter.

Those who feel that their caregiving is inadequate must confront and accept their limitations and acknowledge that these are more than balanced by the loving care they provide. Those who feel guilty about negative feelings toward their spouse can be helped to accept those feelings as natural, understand that the negative feelings do not cancel the positive ones, and forgive themselves for their human reaction to a difficult situation.

Caregivers who blame themselves for their spouses' illness present the greatest difficulty for intervention. These beliefs often prove resistant to change because they are based on well-established personal traits such as a tendency to assume responsibility and control. In this situation professional counseling is probably appropriate.

THE TERMINAL PHASE

For many, the terminal phase of the dying process can be a time of healing. When death is inevitable the need to fight is lifted, releasing energy for reconciliation and preparation. Decisions to be made during this time relate less to treatment and more to ensuring an appropriate and dignified death for the patient. If possible the patient should make these decisions. As Weisman (1972) pointed out, "appropriate death for one person might be unsuitable for another." Families confront several decisions during this time.

Decisions

The patient and family will need to make decisions about where the person will die. Many, but not all, deaths occur in a hospital. This has the advantage of round-the-clock professional support for pain control and symptom management, but may inhibit personal closeness. Further, concerns about liability may lead hospital personnel to use measures to extend life that the family and patient would otherwise reject. Use of a living will (see Chapter 7) may increase the patient's and family's ability to control this situation. Many families decide to keep a dying patient at home despite anxiety about what the death will be like. These anxieties can be allayed to some extent by discussing what families might expect of the death experience. See Leming and Dickinson (1990), *Understanding Dying,* for information about the signs and symptoms of approaching death. The services of a hospice may be used to support home care of a dying person.

Patients and/or families also will need to decide whether to delay the dying process. The patient's decision may be formally expressed in the living will mentioned above. Despite objections and resistance from many medical, legal, and ecclesiastical authorities, many patients choose to hasten their deaths, either by refusing treatment or by committing suicide. An in-depth exploration of this topic is clearly beyond the scope of this work. The interested reader will find excellent discussion of the topic in the books listed in the resource section of this chapter. Further information can be obtained from the Society for the Right to Die (also listed in the "Resources" at the end of this chapter).

Reconciliation

The word "reconcile" has several meanings: to become resigned; to make peace; to adjust or compose. Reconciliation in the face of death has aspects of each. Both caregiver and patient can become resigned to the inevitability of death. On one level, resignation is impossible. As Marion Humphrey pointed out, it is almost impossible to comprehend being a nonperson: "Just as one cannot look at the sun without looking away, we cannot look at our nonbeing without looking away" (1986, p. 67). Although it is almost impossible to conceive of not being, many dying patients and their caregivers can come to accept and prepare for death itself (see Kubler-Ross & Warshaw, 1978, for case studies that illustrate this process).

"Making peace" is crucial to reconciliation. Both patient and caregiver may need to take care of "unfinished business," making amends for past mistakes, letting go of ancient resentments, and saying goodbye. The use of reminiscence will help this process. But making peace need not depend on conversation. Many caregivers find it helpful to keep a journal of their unfinished business. Some of the material in the journal is later discussed with the patient and some is not. Simply acknowledging these burdens can be beneficial. Bloomfield's book *Making Peace with Your Parents* has helpful ideas about taking care of unfinished business.

Preparation

In preparing for a death there are many practical details to take care of and emotional concerns to be addressed. But one is never entirely prepared for the event itself. Still, addressing the details, both practical and emotional, will help ease the transition, freeing energy for the unanticipated.

Practical details. Caregivers will want to know where to find important documents and assets. In preparing for the death it may help to sit down and

Table 9.1

Things to Be Done After a Death Occurs

1. Arrange for members of family or close friends to take turns answering the door or phone, keeping a careful record of calls.

2. Coordinate supplying of food for the next days.

3. Arrange appropriate child care.

4. Decide on time and place of the funeral or any memorial services.

5. If flowers are to be omitted, decide on appropriate memorial to which gifts may be made (such as a church, library, school, or some charity) .

6. Make a list of immediate family, close friends, and employer or business colleagues and notify each by phone.

7. Prepare a list of distant persons to be notified by letter and/or printed notice, and decide which to send to each.

8. Write an obituary and check the cost of placing it in a newspaper or newspapers. Some newspapers charge as much as $200 or more for death notices. In this case, a written notice may be mailed to friends. If you submit a death notice to the paper, include age, place of birth, cause of death, occupation, college degrees, memberships held, military service, outstanding work, and list of survivors in the immediate family; give time and place of services, and deliver it in person, or by phone to newspapers.

9. Arrange hospitality for visiting relatives and friends.

10. Consider special needs of the household, such as cleaning, etc., which might be done by friends.

11. Select pallbearers and notify them (avoid men with heart or back difficulties, or make them honorary pallbearers).

12. If the deceased was living alone, notify utilities and his or her landlord and tell the post office where to send mail. (Take precaution against thieves, especially during the time of the funeral or memorial service.)

13. Plan for disposition of flowers after the funeral (e.g., to a hospital or rest home).

14. Prepare a list of persons to receive acknowledgments of flowers, calls, and so on, and send appropriate acknowledgments (written notes, printed acknowledgments, or some of each).

15. Notify a lawyer and/or the executor and get several copies of the death certificate.

16. Check carefully all life and casualty insurance and death benefits, including any from Social Security, credit union, trade union, fraternal organizations, and military service; also check on income for survivors from these sources.

17. Check promptly on all debts and installment payments. (Some may carry clauses that will cancel them if payments are late. If there is to be a delay in meeting payments, consult with creditors and ask for more time before the payments are due.)

SOURCE: E. Morgan (1988). Dealing Creatively with Death: A Manual of Death Education and Simple Burial. Burnsville, NC Celo.

prepare a list of their locations. Documents will include a will, any living will, insurance policies (including life insurance, health insurance, home insurance), contracts, mortgages, and personal notes. Assets include bank accounts, certificates of deposit, stocks and bonds, and real property. To ensure access to these the caregiver will need to know the location of safe deposit boxes, and names of insurance representatives, lawyers, and brokers.

Many funeral arrangements also can be made in advance. The dying person may want to participate in decisions regarding the funeral or memorial service, possibly to the extent of planning the service and preparing a guest list. Table 9.1 presents a list of things to be done after a death occurs. A more comprehensive listing is offered in *Grief: Climb Toward Understanding,* by Phyllis Davies (1989). Some of these things also can be done in advance.

Emotional preparation. Again, there is no way completely to prepare emotionally for a death, but there are things that can be done to ease the transition for the dying person and the family. These include writing a legacy and anticipating bereavement.

Writing a legacy. People who are dying often need assurance that their life has had meaning. One way to provide this assurance is to prepare a written legacy. This might be organized as a biography, with emphasis on the contributions the person has made. The process of preparing the legacy offers an opportunity for reminiscence as well as reconciliation. Once completed, it can be shared with family members and friends, who may want to add their thoughts on how the person has affected their lives. This legacy can be a gift to both the dying person and survivors—testimony to the value of the life that is ending.

Anticipating mourning. Information about how people often grieve will help caregivers to anticipate their reactions. The most common immediate response to a death, whether it was anticipated or not, is shock, numbness, and disbelief. Beverly Raphael (1983) described later reactions:

> The absence of the dead person is everywhere palpable. The home and familiar environs seem full of painful reminders. Grief breaks over the bereaved in waves of distress. There is intense yearning, pining, and longing for the one who has died. The bereaved feels empty inside, as though torn apart or as if the dead person had been torn out of his body. (p. 40)

These reactions may be accompanied by "searching" behaviors— sensing the loved one's presence, dreams in which the dead person appears, and "seeing" the dead person in the street. Many report receiving "visits" from the dead person (Erikson, Erikson, & Kivnick, 1986). These can be healing experiences, bringing consolation and comfort. They can also be frightening, requiring reassurance. (In this context, their objective reality need not be a central concern.)

People often experience confusion, difficulty concentrating, loneliness, depression, anxiety, panic, guilt, and anger. Physical reactions often include shortness of breath, pain in the chest or stomach, digestive problems, and feelings of suffocation. Sleeping and eating problems are common during this time. In this intense grief, people often fear that they are "going crazy" or "losing control." Reassurance that this is not so will support the grief process.

Caregivers also may experience relief with the death of the loved one. They may be glad the person is no longer suffering. They also may be relieved that their arduous task of care is over. These feelings are natural and should be accepted as such, though some caregivers feel guilty at their relief.

The bereaved often wonder how long their mourning will take. Trainers should emphasize that no time limit can be put on the grieving process, but it is likely that grieving will take much longer than anyone anticipates. In some ways, the bereaved will never be the same, and in some ways, mourning will continue indefinitely. Still, they will need assurance that the acute pain experienced with the loss should subside.

Caregivers might anticipate their reactions by considering how they have handled loss in the past. They also may want to examine the extent to which they have grieved past losses. If they have not, the impending loss may bring with it additional grief from the past. In anticipating bereavement, caregivers may want to identify the resources and liabilities in their social networks. In her descriptions of empathetic, supportive, and destructive people, Ann Stearns (1984) provides an approach to this task. One important resource would be the "empathetic person" who, for example,

> does not shock easily, but accepts your human feelings as human feelings; is not embarrassed by your tears; does not regularly give unwanted advice . . . reminds you of your strengths when you forget that you have these strengths within yourself; . . . acknowledges that he or she is human, too, and shares this humanness; . . . may sometimes become impatient or angry with you but doesn't attack your character when telling you so; . . . tells you honestly when

he or she is unable to be with you because of problems or needs of his or her own; is faithful to commitment and promises (pp. 93-94).

A second type of resource person described by Stearns is the "basic care provider," who

> respects your need for privacy without ignoring your need for human contact, . . . does not encourage you in behaviors that are self-destructive . . . volunteers to help out with tasks that are difficult for you to handle alone . . . anticipates days and dates that may be difficult for you and is especially thoughtful on these occasions . . . keeps confidential whatever personal information that you share (pp. 95-96).

Elizabeth Kubler-Ross (1991) offered another perspective on supportive people:

> When we honestly ask ourselves which persons in our lives mean the most to us, we often find that it is those who, instead of giving much advice, solutions, or cures, have chosen rather to share our pain and touch our wounds with a tender and gentle hand. The friend who can be silent with us in a moment of despair and confusion, who can stay with us in an hour of grief and bereavement, who can tolerate not knowing, not curing, not healing, and face with us the reality of our powerlessness . . . that is the friend who cares.

In contrast to supportive people, "destructive people" complicate mourning.

According to Stearns (1984), the destructive person is one who

> tells others things you intended to have kept in confidence . . . tells you stories of tragedy and catastrophe when you are feeling vulnerable . . . continually questions you and your decisions . . . habitually abuses alcohol or other drugs and encourages you to do the same. Labels your feelings or behavior as "sick," "weird," "neurotic," "hysterical," "abnormal," "childish," "stupid," "lazy," "selfish," or "feeling sorry for yourself." (pp. 98-99)

These categories oversimplify human behavior. Clearly no one is entirely empathetic, supportive, or destructive. But some people are primarily sources of understanding and support, while others can be toxic influences when a person is vulnerable. Those anticipating bereavement may want to do an inventory of the people in their support system, making mental notes to avoid those who have the traits identified with the destructive person, and reach out to the empathetic people and basic care providers available to them.

CHOOSING TO GRIEVE, CHOOSING TO LIVE

With acceptance of loss, the caregiver will often face a choice between reinvesting in life and turning away from life. For some, fear of living without the loved one is overwhelming. In this situation depression or withdrawal is not uncommon.

The choice to reinvest does not require a decision to stop grieving. Instead, those who decide to live also decide to grieve. Experiencing the pain of the loss frees them to live in other ways. Caregiver support programs can support this choice, by supporting the self-love that is necessary to make it and by encouraging the self-care that is a manifestation of that love.

In a single chapter it is difficult, if not impossible, to provide in-depth consideration of a topic such as grief. In a sense grief is simple, and training programs can help by acknowledging it and giving care-givers support for grieving. But grief is also complicated, involving many dimensions of a person's being: physical, cognitive, psy-chological, philosophical, and spiritual. Grief is universal—whenever people experience a loss they grieve, yet it is individual—each person grieves in his or her own way. This chapter provides a limited per-spective. For those interested in further, more in-depth exploration, the resources below offer an excellent starting point.

SUGGESTIONS FOR TRAINERS

A session on grief will address the following objectives:

1. enable participants to become more aware of the losses and grief they have already experienced;
2. address the dilemmas encountered by those caring for terminally ill patients and provide one cognitive approach to coping with them;
3. provide information about mourning and some ways of preparing for death; and

4. prepare for closure by encouraging participants to commit themselves to a personal care program.

Throughout the training, participants have been working to improve their ability to provide care. Self-care has also been a theme. The leader's role during this final session must be to solidify the caregivers' commitment to self-care. I described this commitment as "choosing to live."

During this session, caregivers are encouraged to acknowledge the losses that they are now grieving and prepare for the anticipated loss of their loved one. The dilemmas they encounter when providing care in the face of death should be discussed. Discussion might begin with caregivers identifying dilemmas, which are seen as competing values or "either-or" situations. Using the dilemmas generated by participants, leaders can discuss ways of reframing the dilemmas, replacing the word "or" with the word "and." "Losses and changes are viewed as small deaths.

The "letting go" exercise (see Appendix B) supports caregivers' recognition of the symbolic losses they have and will encounter. Caregivers are encouraged to give themselves permission and support for the current grieving, and to obtain information in preparation for bereavement. Massage can be used as a relaxation exercise. It is best reserved for this last session because people have reservations about massaging people whom they do not know. Because it is so pleasant, massage is a good way to close the training experience.

RESOURCES

Books

Duda, D. (1984). *Coming home: A guide to home care for the terminally ill.* New Mexico: John Muir Publications.

Kalish, R. (1981). *Death, grief, and caring relationships.* Monterey, CA: Brooks/Cole.

Kubler-Ross, E. (1969). *On death and dying.* New York: Macmillan.

Kushner, H. (1981). *When bad things happen to good people.* New York: Schocken.

Lund, D. A. (Ed.). (1989). *Older bereaved spouses: Research with practical applications.* NY: Hemisphere.

Rando, T. (Ed.). (1986). *Loss and anticipatory grief.* Lexington, MA: Lexington Books.

Rando, T. (1988). *Grieving: How to go on living when someone you love dies*. Lexington, MA: Lexington Books.

Worden, J. W. (1982). *Grief counseling and grief therapy: A handbook for the mental health practitioner*. New York: Springer.

Young, V. (1984). *Working with the dying and grieving*. Davis, CA: International Dialogue Press.

Books on Dealing with Guilt

Freeman, L., & Strean, H. (1986). *Guilt: Letting go*. New York: John Wiley.

Jampolsky, G. (1985). *Good-bye to Guilt: Releasing fear through forgiveness*. New York: Bantam.

Books on the Right to Die Issue

Levine, H. (1986). *Life choices: Confronting the life and death decisions created by modern medicine*. New York: Simon & Schuster.

Macklin, R. (1987). *Mortal choices: Bioethics in today's world*. New York: Pantheon.

Winslade, W., & Wilson-Ross, J. (1986). *Choosing life or death: A guide for patients, families and professionals*. New York: Free Press.

Organizations

Society for the Right to Die
250 West 57th Street
New York, NY 10107

REFERENCES

Adler, R., & Towne, N. (1975). *Looking out, looking in, interpersonal communication.* San Francisco: Rinehart Press.

Alzheimer's Disease Research, (1987). The hardest choice: Selecting a nursing home for an Alzheimer's patient, p. xvi. Fockvill, MA: American Health Assistance Foundation.

Archbold, P. G. (1982). An analysis of parentcaring by women. *Home Health Care Services Quarterly, 3*(2), 5-26.

Baltes, M. M., & Baltes, P. B. (Eds.). (1986). *The psychology of control and aging.* Hillsdale, NJ: Lawrence Erlbaum.

Bandura, A. (1977). Self-efficacy: Toward a unifying theory of behavioral change. *Psychological Review, 84,* 191-215.

Barusch, A. S. (1987). Power dynamics in the aging family: A preliminary statement. *Journal of Gerontological Social Work, 11*(3/4), 43-57.

Barusch, A. S. (1988). Problems and coping strategies of elderly spouse caregivers. *The Gerontologist, 28,* 677-685.

Barusch, A. S., & Miller, L. S. (1986). The effect of services on family assistance to the frail elderly. *Journal of Social Service Research, 9*(1), 31-45.

Barusch, A. S., & Spaid, W. M. (1989). Gender differences in caregiving: Why do wives report greater burden? *The Gerontologist, 29,* 667-676.

Barusch, A. S., & Spaid, W. M. (in press). Reducing caregiver burden through short-term training: Evaluation findings from a caregiver support project. *Journal of Gerontological Social Work.*

Barusch, A. S., Zhang, M., Wu, W., Jin, H., & Cai, G. (in press). Intergenerational relations in contemporary China: Descriptive findings from Shanghai. In H. Sheppard (Ed.), *Proceedings of the Second International Conference on Aging and Social Policies in Asia and the U.S.* International Exchange Center for Gerontology, Tampa, Florida.

Beisecker, A. E. (1988). Aging and the desire for information and input in medical decisions: Patient consumerism in medical encounters. *The Gerontologist, 28* (3), 330-335.

Beisecker, A. E. (1989). *Health promotion and support for caregivers: A survey of programs targeting the rural elderly.* Unpublished manuscript.

Bell, R. (1981). *Worlds of friendship*. Beverly Hills, CA: Sage.

Bloomfield, H. (1984). *Making peace with your parents*. New York: Ballantine.

Boss, G., & Seegmiller, J. E. (1981). Age-related physiological changes and their clini significance. *Western Journal of Medicine, 135*, 13-19.

Bower, S. A., & Bower, G. H. (1984). *Asserting yourself: A practical guide for positive chan* Reading, MA: Addison-Wesley.

Bradburn, N. M. (1969). *The structure of psychological well-being*. Chicago: University Chicago Press.

Brahce, C. I. (1983). Creating partnerships with family caretakers. In M. A. Smyer & M. G (Eds.), *Mental health and aging*. Beverly Hills, CA: Sage.

Branch, L. G., & Jette, A. M. (1983). Elders' use of long-term care assistance. *The Gerontolog: 23*, 51-56.

Brody, E. M. (1981). Women in the middle. *The Gerontologist, 27*, 471-480.

Bronfenbrenner, U. (1979). *The ecology of human development*. Cambridge, MA: Harva University Press.

Bruning, J. L., & Kintz, B. L. (1968). *Computational handbook of statistics*. Glenview, IL: Scc Foresman.

Buckalew, M. W. (1982). *Learning to control stress* (2nd. ed.). New York: Richard Rosen Pre:

Bugental, J. (1973). Confronting the existential meaning of my death through exercis *Interpersonal Development, 4*, 148-163.

Campbell, R., & Brody, E. (1985). Women's changing roles and help to the elderly: Attitud of women in the United States and Japan. *The Gerontologist, 25*, 584-592.

Cantor, M. H. (1983). Strain among caregivers: A study of experience in the United States. *T. Gerontologist, 23*(6), 597-604.

Cicirelli, V. G. (1981). *Helping elderly parents: The role of adult children*. Boston: Auburn Hous

Colgrove, M. (1981). *How to survive the loss of a love: Fifty-eight things to do when there nothing to be done*. New York: Bantam.

Cowley, M. (1982). *The view from 80*. New York: Penquin.

Cunningham, W. R., & Owens, W. A. (1983). The Iowa state study of the adult development intellectual abilities. In K. W. Schaie (Ed.), *Longitudinal studies of adult psychologic: development*. New York: Guilford Press.

Davies, P. (1989). *Grief: Climb toward understanding*. New York: Carol Publishing Group.

Dawson, D., Hendershot, G., & Fulton, J. (1987). *Aging in the eighties: Functional limitatio of individuals age 65 years and over* (Vital and Health Statistics, No. 133, June 10 Washington, DC: National Center for Health Statistics.

Derogatis, L., & Spencer, P. M. (1982). *The Brief Symptom Inventory (BSI): Administration ar procedures manual*. Baltimore: Clinical Psychometric Research Unit, Johns Hopkins Un versity School of Medicine.

Eagles, J. M., Beattie, J. A. G., Blackwood, G. W., Restall, D. B., & Ashcroft, G. W. (1987 The mental health of elderly couples, 1. The effects of a cognitively impaired spouse. *Britis Journal of Psychiatry, 150*, 299-303.

Eastwood, H. D. H. (1972). Bowel transit studies in the elderly. *Gerontology Clinician, 1: 154-160.

Ellis, A. (1975). *How to live with a "neurotic" at home and at work*. New York: Crowne.

Erikson, E., Erikson, J., & Kivnick, H. Q. (1986). *Vital involvement in old age*. New Yor| Norton.

Fallcreek, S., & Mettler, M. (1983). A healthy old age: A sourcebook for health promotion wi: older adults (rev. ed.). *Journal of Gerontological Social Work, 6*, 2/3.

Felder, L. (1990). *When a loved one is ill: How to take better care of your loved one, your family, and yourself*. New York: New American Library.

Fengler, A. P., & Goodrich, P. (1979). Wives of elderly men: The hidden patients. *The Gerontologist, 19*(2), 175-183.

Fitting, M. D., & Rabins, P. (1985, Fall). Men and women: Do they give care differently? *Generations, 23-26.*

Frankfather, D. L. (1981). Provider discretion and consumer preference in long-term care for seriously disabled elderly. *The Gerontologist, 21*(4), 366-373.

Freeman, L., & Strean, H. (1986). *Guilt: Letting go*. New York: John Wiley.

Fromm, E. (1956). *The art of loving*. New York: Bantam.

Gallagher, D. (1987). Assessing affect in the elderly. *Clinics in Geriatric Medicine, 3*(1), 65-85.

Gallagher, D., Rose, J., Rivera, P., Lovett, S., & Thompson, L. W. (1989). Prevalence of depression in family caregivers. *The Gerontologist, 29,* 449-456.

Gambrill, E. D., & Richey, C. A. (1975). An assertion inventory for use in assessment and research. *Behavior Therapy, 6,* 550-561.

Goldfried, M. R. (1980). Psychotherapy as coping skills training. In M. J. Mahoney (Ed.), *Psychotherapy process: Current issues and future directions*. New York: Plenum.

Greene, V. L., & Monahan, D. J. (1987). The effect of a professionally guided caregiver support and education group on institutionalization of care receivers. *The Gerontologist, 27,* 716-721.

Hooyman, N. R., & Kiyak, H. A. (1988). *Social gerontology: A multidisciplinary perspective*. Boston: Allyn & Bacon.

Humphrey, M. A. (1986). Effects of anticipatory grief for the patient, family member, and caregiver. In T. A. Rando (Ed.) *Loss and anticipatory grief,* pp. 63-79. Lexington, MA: Lexington Books.

Jaloweic, A., Murphy, S., & Powers, M. (1984). Psychometric assessment of the Jaloweic Coping Scale. *Nursing Research, 33,* 157-161.

Jencks, B. (1980, July). *Handling stress in the work setting*. Paper presented at the meeting of the Utah Perinatal Association.

Johnson, C., & Catalano, D. J. (1981). Childless elderly and their family supports. *The Gerontologist, 21*(6), 610-618.

Kaye, L., & Applegate, J. (1990). *Men as caregivers to the elderly: Understanding and aiding unrecognized family support*. Lexington, MA: Lexington Books.

Kemper, D. W., Mettler, M., Guiffre, J., & Matzek, B. (1986). *Growing wiser: The older person's guide to mental wellness*. Boise, ID: Healthwise.

Kemper, P. R., Applebaum, R., & Harrigan, M. (1987). Community care demonstrations: What have we learned? *Health Care Financing Review, 8*(4), 87-100.

Kinney, J. M., & Stephens, M. A. P. (1989). Hassles and uplifts of giving care to a family member with dementia. *Psychology and Aging, 4*(4), 402-408.

Kiresuk, T. J., & Lund, S. H. (1978). Goal attainment scaling. In C. C. Attkinsson, W. A. Hargreaves, M. J. Horowitz, & J. E. Sorensen (Eds.), *Evaluation of human service programs* (pp. 341-370). New York: Academic Press.

Kosburg, J. I., & Cairl, R. E. (1986). The Cost of Care Index: A case management tool for screening informal care providers. *The Gerontologist, 26*(3), 273-278.

Krause, N. (1986). Stress and coping: Reconceptualizing the role of locus of control beliefs. *Journal of Gerontology, 41,* 617-622.

Krout, J. A. (1986). *The Aged in Rural America*. New York: Greenwood Press.

Kubler-Ross, E. (1991, January 29). Personal communication.

Kubler-Ross, E. (1969). *On Death and Dying.* New York: Macmillan.

Kubler-Ross, E., & Warshaw, M. (1978). *To live until we say good-bye.* Englewood Cliffs, NJ: Prentice-Hall.

Kushner, H. (1981). *When bad things happen to good people.* New York: Schocken.

Lazarus, R. S., & Folkman, S. (1984). *Stress, appraisal, and coping.* New York: Springer.

Leming, M. R., & Dickinson, G. E. (1990). *Understanding dying, death, & bereavement* (2nd. ed.). Troy, MO: Holt, Rinehart & Winston.

Liang, J., & Tu, E. J. (1986). Estimating lifetime risk of nursing home residency: A further note. *The Gerontologist, 26*(5), 560-563.

Litwak, E. (1985). *Helping the elderly.* New York: Guilford Press.

Lopata, H. Z. (1978). Contributions of extended families to the support systems of metropolitan area widows: Limitations of the modified kin networks. *Journal of Marriage and Family, 40,* 355-364.

Lorensen, M. (1985). Effects on elderly women's self-care in case of acute hospitalization as compared with men. *Health Care for Women International, 6,* 247-265.

Lubben, J. E. (1988). Assessing social networks among elderly populations. *Family and Community Health, 11,* 42-52.

Lund, D. A., Dimond, M. F., Caserta, M. S., Johnson, R. J., Poulton, J. L., & Connelly, J. R. (1985/1986). Identifying elderly with coping difficulties after two years of bereavement. *Omega, 16*(3). 213-224.

Lund, D. A., Pett, M. A., & Caserta, M. S.(1987). Institutionalizing dementia victims: Some caregiver considerations. *Journal of Gerontological Social Work, 11,* 119-135.

Mace, N. L., & Rabins, P. V. (1981). *The 36-hour day: A family guide to caring for persons with Alzheimer's disease, related dementing illnesses, and memory loss in later life.* Baltimore, MA: Johns Hopkins University Press.

Mangen, D. J., & Peterson, W. A. (Eds.). (1982). *Research instruments in social gerontology: Social roles and social participation* (Vol. 2). Minneapolis: University of Minnesota Press.

Mathews, S. H. (1986). *Friendships through the life course: Oral biographies in old age.* Beverly Hills, CA: Sage.

McCubbin, H., Larsen, A., & Olson, D. (1981). F-COPES (Family Crisis-Oriented Personal Evaluation Scales). St. Paul, MN: University of Minnesota, Family Social Science.

Meichenbaum, D., & Jaremko, M. E. (Eds.). (1983). *Stress reduction and prevention.* New York: Plenum.

Milardo, R. M. (1983). Social networks and pair relationships: A review of substantive and measurement issues. *Sociology and Social Research, 68,* 1-18.

Montgomery, R. J. V., & Borgatta, E. F. (1989). The effects of alternative support strategies on family caregiving. *The Gerontologist, 29,* 457-464.

Montgomery, R. J. V., Gonyea, J. G., & Hooyman, N. R. (1985). Caregiving and the experience of subjective and objective burden. *Family Relations, 34,* 19-26.

Morgan, E. (Ed.). (1988). *Dealing creatively with death: A manual of death education and simple burial.* Burnsville, NC: Cleo Press.

National Center for Health Statistics. (1972). *Home care for persons 55 and over, U.S., July 1966-June 1968* (Vital and Health Statistics, Series 10, No. 73, DHEW Publication No. HSM72-1062). Washington, DC: Government Printing Office.

Nelson, G. (1980). Social services to the urban and rural aged: The experience of Area Agencies on Aging. *The Gerontologist, 20,* 200-207.

Neuber, K. A., & Associates. (1980). *Needs assessment: A model for community planning.* Beverly Hills, CA: Sage.

Norusis, M. J. (1986). *Advanced Statistics SPSS/PC+ for the IBM PC/XT/AT*. Chicago: SPSS.

Olson, D. H., McCubbin, H. I., Barnes, H., Larsen, A., Muxen, M., & Wilson, M. (1983). *Families: What makes them work*. Beverly Hills, CA: Sage.

Owens, W. A. (1966). Age and mental abilities: A second adult follow-up. *Journal of Educational Psychology, 57*, 311-325.

Pagel, M. D., Becker, J., & Coppel, D. B. (1985). Loss of control, self-blame and depression: An investigation of spouse caregivers of Alzheimer's disease patients. *Journal of Abnormal Psychology, 94*, 169-182.

Palmore, E. (1983). Health care needs of the rural elderly. *International Journal of Aging and Human Development, 18*, 39-45.

Palmore, E. (1976). Total chance of institutionalization among the aged. *The Gerontologist, 16*(6), 504-507.

Parkes, C. M., & Weiss, R. S. (1983). *Recovery from bereavement*. New York: Basic Books.

Pattison, E. M. (1977). (Ed.). *The experience of dying*. Englewood Cliffs, NJ: Prentice-Hall.

Peale, N. V. (1956). *The power of positive thinking*. Englewood Cliffs, NJ: Prentice-Hall.

Pratt, C., Schmall, V., Wright, S., & Cleland, M. (1985). Burden and coping strategies of caregivers to Alzheimer's disease patients. *Family Relations, 34*, 27-34.

Quinn, M. J., & Tomita, S. K. (1986). *Elderly abuse and neglect: Assessment and intervention*. New York: Springer.

Raphael, B. (1983). *The anatomy of bereavement*. New York: Basic Books.

Rando, T. (1986). Understanding and facilitating anticipatory grief in the loved ones of the dying. In T. Rando (Ed.), *Loss and anticipatory grief* (pp. 97-131). Lexington, MA: Lexington Books.

Reeder, L. G. (1972). The patient-client as a consumer: Some observations on the changing professional-client relationship. *Journal of Health and Social Behavior, 13*, 406-412.

Robinson, B., & Thurnher, M. (1979). Taking care of aged parents: A family life cycle transition. *The Gerontologist, 19*(6), 586-593.

Schaie, K. W., & Strother, C. R. (1968). A cross-sequential study of age changes in cognitive behavior. *Psychological Bulletin, 70*, 671-680.

Seligman, M. E. P. (1975). *Helplessness: On depression, development and death*. San Francisco: W. H. Freeman.

Shanas, E. (1980). Older people and their families: The new pioneers. *Journal of Marriage and the Family, 42*(1), 9-15.

Shanas, E. (1979). The family as a support system in old age. *The Gerontologist, 19*(2), 169-174.

Siegel, B. S. (1989). *Peace, love and healing*. New York: Harper & Row.

Silverman, P. (1974). Anticipatory grief from the perspective of widowhood. In B. Schoenberg, A. Carr, A. Kutscher, D. Peretz, & I. Goldberg (Eds.), *Anticipatory grief* (pp. 320-330). New York: Columbia University Press.

Sirrocco, A. (1989). Nursing home characteristics: 1986 inventory of long-term care places (Vital Health Statistics, Series 14, No. 33). Washington, DC: National Center for Health Statistics.

Skinner, B. F., & Vaughn, M. E. (1983). *Enjoy old age: Living fully in your later years*. New York: Warner Books.

Sloan, R. W. (1986). *Practical geriatric therapeutics*. Oradell, NJ: Medical Economics Books.

Smith, M. J. (1987). *When I say no I feel guilty*. New York: Bantam.

Spaid, W. M., & Barusch, A. S. (in press). Social support and caregiver strain: The impact of positive and aversive social contacts on elderly spouse caregivers. *Journal of Gerontological Social Work*.

Stearns, A. K. (1984). *Living through personal crisis.* Chicago: Thomas More Press.

Stone, R., Cafferata, G. L., & Sangl, J. (1987). Caregivers of the frail elderly: A national profile. *The Gerontologist, 27,* 616-626.

Strain, L., & Chappell, N. (1982). Confidants. *Research on Aging, 4,* 479-502.

Sussman, M. (1955). The help pattern in the middle-class family. In M. Sussman (Ed.), *Sourcebook in marriage and the family* (pp. 304-310). Boston: Houghton Mifflin.

Tate, L. A., & Brennan, C. M. (1988). *Adult day care: A practical guidebook and manual.* New York: Haworth.

Toseland, R. W., & Rossiter, C. M. (1989). Group interventions to support family caregivers: A review and analysis. *The Gerontologist, 29,* 438-448.

Toseland, R. W., Rossiter, C. M., & Labrecque, M. S. (1989a). The effectiveness of peer-led and professionally led groups to support family caregivers. *The Gerontologist, 29,* 465-471.

Toseland, R. W., Rossiter, C. M., & Labrecque, M. S. (1989b). The effectiveness of three group intervention strategies to support family caregivers. *American Journal of Orthopsychiatry, 59*(3), 420-429.

Toseland, R. W., & Zarit, S. H. (1989). Group interventions to support family caregivers: A review and analysis. *The Gerontologist, 29,* 438-448.

Uhlenberg, P. (1979). Older women: The growing challenge to design constructive roles. *The Gerontologist, 19*(3), 236-241.

U.S. Bureau of the Census. (1976). Demographic aspects of aging and the older population in the United States (Current Population Reports, Series P-23, No. 59). Washington, DC: Government Printing Office.

U.S. Bureau of the Census. (1982). *Projections of the population of the United States: 1982-2050* (Current Population Reports, Series P-25, No. 922). Washington, DC: Government Printing Office.

U.S. Bureau of the Census. (1989). *Statistical abstract of the United States: 1989* (109th ed.). Washington, DC: Government Printing Office.

U.S. Senate Special Committee on Aging. (1986). *Aging America: Trends and projections* (1985-1986 ed.). Washington, DC: Department of Health and Human Services.

Ward, R. (1978). Limitations of the family as a supportive institution in the lives of the aged. *The Family Coordinator,* 365-372.

Ward, R. (1985). Informal networks and well-being in later life: A research agenda. *The Gerontologist, 25,* 55-61.

Watson, R. R. (1985). CRC handbook of nutrition in the aged. Boca Raton, FL: CRC Press.

Weisman, A. D. (1972). *On dying and denying: A psychiatric study of terminality.* New York: Behavioral Publications.

West, G. E., & Simons, R. L. (1983). Sex differences in stress, coping, resources, and illness among the elderly. *Research on Aging, 5,* 253-268.

Westbrook, M. T., & Viney, L. I. (1983). Age and sex differences in patients' reactions to illness. *Journal of Health and Social Behavior, 24,* 313-324.

Wright, S. D., Lund, D. A., Caserta, M., & Pratt, C. (in press). Coping and caregiver well-being: The impact of maladaptive strategies. *Journal of Gerontological Social Work.*

Zarit, S. H., Orr, N. K., & Zarit, J. M. (1985). *The hidden victims of Alzheimer's disease.* New York: New York University Press.

Zarit, S. H., Reever, K. E., & Bach-Peterson, J. (1980). Relatives of the impaired elderly: Correlates of feelings of burden. *The Gerontologist, 20,* 651-656.

Zarit, S. H., & Toseland, R. W. (1989). Current and future direction in family caregiving research. *The Gerontologist, 29,* 481-483.

APPENDIX A : Evaluation of the University of Utah Caregiver Support Program

The University of Utah's Caregiver Support Project (CSP) was established in 1986, with funding from the Administration on Aging (OHDS Grant No. 90AM0221). Its goal was to develop and evaluate interventions to reduce the stress experienced by an elderly caregiver. The original *Wellsprings* intervention consisted of six different 2-hour sessions. Topics discussed included ageism and its impact on the older caregiver; healthy relationships; healthy physical aging; community resources; legal and financial issues; grief; and self-care. In addition to these, I have added a session on caregiving skills, so the program presented here consists of seven sessions. The sessions emphasize development of personal coping and interpersonal communication skills. A variety of techniques to relieve stress, such as relaxation exercises, massage, and visualization are described.

CSP Participants

A total of 140 caregivers participated in the CSP program. They were primarily (95%) white. The majority (70%) were women. Caregivers averaged 70 years of age, and had been providing care for an average of 66 months. The average length of marriage was 39 years. Participants generally reported an annual household income between $10,001 and $15,000 per year.

Care receivers averaged 73 years of age. Half (53%) had a primary diagnosis of dementia. Other diagnoses included stroke, Parkinson's disease, lung disease, and general frailty. Of a total of seven possible activities of daily living (bathing, dressing, transfer, toileting, continence care, feeding, and walking) care recipients required assistance or supervision with an average of 4.3 of them.

CSP Evaluation

In order to evaluate the program, pre- and post-interviews were conducted, as well as a final follow-up interview completed six months after the training. Ninety-five caregivers completed all the interviews. The evaluation design compared four training conditions as presented in Table A.1.

Caregivers were randomly assigned to either the family-participation condition or the individual condition. In the family-participation condition, caregivers were directed to bring a family member with them to sessions. In the individual condition, they were instructed to come alone. The in-home format was developed for caregivers who were unable or unwilling to attend group meetings. This format was similar in that it involved six weekly sessions based on the *Wellsprings* curriculum. Unlike group participants, in-home caregivers were rarely assigned to the family-participation condition. One reflection of the isolation experienced by these caregivers is the lack of significant others to participate in training. In-home caregivers were often unable to arrange for a family member to join them in training. In this case they were reassigned to the individual condition, in order to maintain the integrity of the family-participation approach. In-home training was provided by an MSW with specialized preparation in gerontology, while group training was provided by a team of two leaders, one MSW and one MED.

Detailed findings from the CSP evaluation are presented in an article soon to appear in the *Journal of Gerontological Social Work* (Barusch & Spaid, in press). Results suggested the *Wellsprings* intervention improved coping effectiveness, increased active coping, and slightly reduced caregiver burden. The intervention was associated with an 18% average gain in overall coping effectiveness, as well as a significant decline in the proportion of problems that overwhelmed the caregivers. This was seen as a 47% drop in the percentage of problems with which they failed to cope. We also observed a 21% in-

Table A.1
Training Conditions

| | | Training Condition | | |
	Individual Caregivers		Family-Participation	
Training Location	Group	$n = 37$	$n = 33$	Subtotal = 70
	In-home	$n = 22$	$n = 3$	Subtotal = 25
	Subtotal = 59		Subtotal = 36	Total = 95

crease in the percentage of problem situations that caregivers changed through personal action. Despite declines in patient functional status, caregivers also reported lower levels of subjective and objective burden following training. Overall changes were small, amounting to a 4% decline in subjective burden and a 7% drop in objective burden. Family participation in group training sessions enhanced the impact of the intervention.

APPENDIX B: Exercises

This appendix presents exercises for relaxation and effective communication. When a training program involves weekly meetings, the trainer may want to combine one relaxation and one communication exercise in each week's curriculum.

RELAXATION TECHNIQUES

Do not expect relaxation exercises to help motivate you or to make you want to do something. Relaxation is not a motivational technique. Instead, it is designed to help you cope with anxiety and tension. It is intended to reduce the tension that keeps you from acting the way you would like or leads you to feel bad about yourself. From the wide array of relaxation techniques that are available, I have chosen seven distinct approaches that seem well-suited to the needs of family caregivers. For more, see the resource list at the end of this chapter.

How to relax. Several psychologists have written about methods for relaxation. Some are based on muscle relaxation techniques and breathing, others rely on visual imagery, still others are based on "talking yourself" into relaxation.

Relaxation Technique 1: Deep Breathing

When most of us are asked to take a deep breath our chests go up and spread out. This type of breathing does not reduce tension. In fact, it can increase our feelings of stress. Abdominal breathing, on the other hand, reduces stress. To practice abdominal breathing, place your hands on your stomach, low on the abdomen. Then inhale, pretending that your mouth is around a straw. Exhale, making a hissing sound. During the next inhalation, count to five slowly—hold your breath for about 2 seconds, and then exhale for 10 counts. Some who use this technique suggest that the inhale and exhale have different effects. Focusing on an inhale may help to muster up courage, strength, or energy. Focusing on the exhale may help to push things away, to relieve stress.

Deep Breathing

1. Sit upright in a comfortable position. Keep your back straight, your feet flat on the floor, and your hand on your abdomen.
2. Inhale, pretending your mouth is around a straw. Breathe slowly, inhaling until it is almost impossible to take in more air. Your abdomen should expand against your hands. (Count to five as you inhale.)
3. Hold your breath for a count of two.
4. Exhale slowly, making a hissing sound while you breath out all the air in your lungs. (Count to 10 as you exhale.)
5. Pause for a second and repeat the process.

If you should become dizzy while practicing deep breathing, pause for several seconds and breathe normally before repeating the process.

Relaxation Technique 2: Muscle Relaxation

The purpose of muscle relaxation is to experience the difference between tension and relaxation in your muscles. This is done through a series of exercises designed to help you experience this difference.

Sit or lie in as comfortable a position as you can. Make sure that your legs and arms are uncrossed. Remove or loosen any article of clothing that causes you even a slight amount of discomfort. If you wear contact lenses, it would be best to remove them. It also would be best to do these exercises alone unless others in the room are serious about learning how to relax and will do the exercises with you. While you are in this comfortable position, read the following relaxation instructions without doing them.

> Clench both fists tightly as if you were squeezing all the juice out of an imaginary orange in each hand. Notice the muscles in your fingers and lower forearm—they are tight, tense, pulling. Clench your fists like this for about 5 seconds, then relax—just let your fists go. Drop the imaginary orange in each hand. Pay attention to the sensations you now have in the muscles of your fingers, hands, and forearms as they relax. There is a sort of flow of relaxation—perhaps a kind of warmth—in those muscles. Notice and enjoy this relaxation for about 20 or 30 seconds. Okay, clench your fists again, tightly. Notice the tension, especially from your fingers and lower forearms. Now relax, let go—just allow the muscles to loosen. The relaxation is not something you make happen, but something you allow to happen. Notice the difference between tension and relaxation in those muscles.

Repeat this procedure a third time.

> Now, reach out in front of you with both arms, stretch forward with your arms like a lazy tomcat. Move your extended arms over your head, reach for the sky, and hold it. Now, stretch yours arms out to the sides, back to the overhead position, again out in front of you, and let your arms drop to your lap. Allow the arms to relax. Again, feel the release of tension, this time in the muscles of your upper arms, shoulders, and upper back. Enjoy the lack of tension in the muscles as they become more relaxed, then still more relaxed, and more relaxed than ever before.

Repeat this procedure again until your upper arms, shoulders, and extreme upper back are completely relaxed. This usually takes from two to four times, as do most muscle relaxation exercises.

Add the other muscle relaxation exercises one at a time. The list below tells you which muscles to tighten and relax for each exercise. Remember that each time you do an exercise you should tense the muscle for about 5 seconds and then let go completely with that muscle group, experiencing the contrasting relaxation for 20 to 30 seconds. Repeat each exercise three times during each relaxation period (a relaxation session will last about 20 minutes). In order to obtain maximum results, you should spend at least one session per day relaxing. The more practice you get in muscle relaxation, the easier it will become to control your anxiety in every day life. The suggested muscle groups that need to be relaxed during each session are listed below. Do not do any exercises yet. Just read the list and become familiar with it.

Muscle Relaxation Exercises

Muscle Area	*Instructions*	*Tension Location*
Hands	Clench and relax both fists.	The back of your hands and your wrists
Upper arms	Bend your elbows and fingers of both hands to your shoulders and biceps muscles. Relax.	The biceps muscle
Lower arms	Hold both arms straight out and stretch. Relax.	The upper portion of forearms
Forehead	Wrinkle your forehead and raise your eyebrows. Relax.	The entire forehead area
Forehead	Frown and lower your eyebrows. Relax.	The lower part of the forehead, especially in the region between the eyes.
Eyes	Close your eyes tightly. Relax.	The eyelids
Jaws	Clench your jaws tightly. Relax.	The jaws and cheeks
Tongue	Bring your tongue upward and press it against the roof of your mouth. Feel tension. Relax.	The area in and around the tongue
Mouth	Press your lips lightly together. Feel tension. Relax.	The region around the mouth

Neck	Press your head backward. Roll to the right, shift roll to left, and straighten. Relax.	The muscles in back of the neck and at the base of the scalp. Right and left sides of neck
Neck and jaw	Bend your head forward, press the chin against the chest. Straighten and relax.	The muscles in front of the neck and around the jaw
Shoulders	Bring your shoulders upward toward your ears, shrug, and move around. Relax.	The muscles of the shoulders and the lower part of the neck
Chest	Take a deep breath and hold it for 5 seconds. Relax.	The entire chest area
Abdomen	Tighten your stomach muscles hard. Relax.	The entire abdominal region
Back	Arch your back from chair. Relax.	Lower back
Thighs	Press your heels down as hard as you can, then flex your thighs.	The muscles in the lower part of the thighs
Legs	Hold both legs out and point your toes away from face. Relax.	The muscles of the calf
Legs	Toes toward face	Muscles below knee cap

Relaxation Technique 3: Crisis Breathing

During a crisis, it is essential that caregivers have their wits about them. One specific technique that can be used to marshall energy and prepare to cope with a crisis is based upon abdominal breathing. The following four steps should be taken before starting to cope with the crisis. First, exhale. This exhale enables you to detach yourself from the situation, to push things away for a moment. Next, inhale slowly and assess the situation. A second exhale is used to relax. And a final inhale will energize you to move forward and cope with the situation.

Crisis Breathing

1. Exhale, distance yourself from the situation.
2. Inhale slowly and assess the situation.
3. Exhale, relax.
4. Inhale, energize.

This exercise is adapted from Jencks (1980).

Relaxation Technique 4: Chinese Breath Exercise

This short breath exercise comes from the Chinese Tai Chi Chuan. Three short inhales are done through the nose (without exhale).

1. Stand with your arms relaxed at your side.
2. On the first inhale, lift arms from the sides straight out in front at shoulder height.
3. On the second inhale, open the arms straight out to the sides, keeping them at shoulder height.
4. On the third inhale, lift the arms straight over the head.
5. On the exhale, through the mouth, move the arms in an arc back to the sides.

This exercise allows the body to lead the mind and spirit to greater openness to others and to the environment.

Relaxation Technique 5: Instant Relaxation (3, 2, 1)

Instant relaxation is another method of achieving relaxation and counteracting the effects of stress. This procedure is quick, easy to learn, requires no time out, and can be practiced as often as you like throughout the day.

Instant relaxation involves mentally sending your muscles a message that signals them to relax. To practice instant relaxation, do the following:

1. Mentally divide your body into three parts. *Part 1* is the legs. *Part 2* is the torso or trunk. *Part 3* consists of your head, neck, shoulders, and arms.

2. Tense *all* muscles.

3. After 10 seconds, say to yourself the number "3" and relax all muscles in your head, neck, shoulders, and arms.

4. After 10 seconds more, say to yourself the number "2" and relax all muscles in your chest, abdomen, and back.

Concentrate on breathing as normally as possible.

5. After 10 seconds more, say to yourself the number "1" and relax all the muscles in your legs.

6. Concentrate on how it feels to be completely relaxed, to have normal breathing, and yet be very alert, energized, and ready to go about the day's activities.

Repeat the above steps six or more times, moving through the steps faster and faster each time. The last practice session should be done as quickly as you can say to yourself "3, 2, 1."

To use this procedure, you just say to yourself "3, 2, 1." You do not have to tense your muscles because they have gradually become tense on their own as you have gone through the day. At this point, you may be wondering how saying the numbers "3, 2, 1" can relax you. This method works because you have associated the various numbers with your different body parts. When you say the number "3" you automatically send your head, neck, shoulders, and arms a message to relax.

Again, this method of relaxation is quick, easy to learn, and can be done at anytime throughout the day. You can use this method before, after, or during stressful situations as a way to staying totally relaxed. If used every day, regularly, instant relaxation can help prevent stress before it occurs and/or minimize its harmful effects.

This exercise is adapted from Buckalew (1982).

Relaxation Technique 6: Visualization

Visualization can be a very effective relaxation exercise. Take three deep breaths to help slow the body down and then use the visualization. In creating the images, use the words as bait and allow your subconscious to change the image if it wants. *Use as many senses as you can: seeing, hearing, tasting, smelling, touching.* This allows the experience to be as "full" as possible. Soft, soothing music played in the background can add to this experience. Then the group leader can read a visualization in a soft voice. Two examples are listed below. For other visualizations, see Bernie S. Siegel's book, *Peace, Love and Healing* (1989) listed in the resource section for this chapter.

1. See a cloud drifting across the sky. Now it is gone. See another and imagine that you are on it drifting up over the city. As you drift and float, you come to a wooded area where you can hear birds chirping and see animals scurrying about. (Pause) You see a stream of water nearby. As you near the water, you notice how gentle, yet consistent the movement of the water is. It is peaceful yet energetic. (Pause) Now move away to a large meadow, and in the meadow we can see wildflowers. Look at the lovely colors. (Pause) And now, begin to drift away from this place, back to the room you are in. (Pause) Take in a slow deep breath, and let it go. Repeat breathing three times, then open your eyes and stretch.

2. Imagine the sun above you. With your imagination, pick a beam of sunlight and direct it to move down to your body. Feel the warm glow as the sun is an energy that helps growth and healing. Take special note to direct this energy to any particular part of the body that feels uncomfortable or ill at ease. (Pause.) Now, select an area of your life that you would like to see grow. Isolate that area and see it as a seed. (Pause.) Direct the sunbeam toward this seed with the knowledge that this energy can help its growth and expansion. Let the sun surround and fill the seed with warmth and light (Pause.) After a few moments, let the image go. Take in a deep breath and let it go. Repeat breathing three times, then open your eyes and stretch.

Relaxation Technique 7: Shoulder and Neck Massage

Have your partner sit comfortably in a chair. Stand behind him or her and suggest that he or she remove glasses, close his or her eyes, and think "I am relaxing."

1. Allow your hands to greet your partner by placing them warmly on his or her shoulders.

2. Apply gentle but firm and even pressure with your thumbs across the top of the shoulders. Work your way toward the neck and then back across to the ends of the shoulders.

3. Using both hands, massage across the top of the shoulders with a kneading motion.

4. Locate the vertebrae at the base of the neck. Place your thumbs on either side of the vertebrae and apply gentle but firm pressure away from the spine. Continue down the back. Do *not* press on the spine itself.

5. Locate the indentations at the base of the skull on either side of the spine at the back of the head. Apply rotating pressure with your thumbs.

6. Stand beside your partner. Place one hand on his or her forehead and one hand behind his or her head for support. *Slowly and carefully* rotate the head first in one direction and then in the other.

7. Stand behind your partner again and use three fingers to massage the jaw area. Have your partner clench his or her jaw. You will easily find the muscles that need to be rubbed!

8. Use fingers to gently massage the temples. Work across the forehead and back to the temples.

9. Bring your hands back to the shoulders and allow your hands to "say good-bye."

How do your feel? Sharing this experience with someone is a warm and caring exchange. It is relaxing for both the giver and the receiver of the massage. Some of the steps (3, 5, 7, and 8) can also be used for self-massage.

This massage sequence is from Fallcreek & Mettler (1983, P. 122).

COMMUNICATION TECHNIQUES

Caregivers can benefit from several communication techniques. Assertiveness will be crucial for those who work with medical and social service providers and can improve relationships within the family as well. Criticism and conflict also pose problems for many caregivers. Assertive communication techniques for coping with criticism and managing conflict are presented in this section. In a training setting, the exercises presented may be done as a group or in dyads. Role plays are often effective for demonstrating these techniques. The Bill of Assertive Rights presented at the end of this appendix may be a useful handout.

Communication Technique 1: Understanding Assertiveness

In order for caregivers to care for themselves and use services to which they are entitled, they need to understand and use assertive communication techniques. Many older people view assertiveness as aggressiveness, thinking the assertive person is "mean" or "insensitive." It is important to clarify the difference between assertive, passive, and aggressive communication. I recommend using the material from the *Growing Wiser* manual (Kemper et al., 1986) developed by Healthwise, Inc., as background for this discussion.

Essentially, assertive communication is standing up for our rights, without violating the rights of others. Passive communication is failing to protect our rights, often because we feel they (and we) are less important than the rights of others. Aggressive communication is fighting for what we want, without consideration for the rights of others. The *Growing Wiser* manual associates passive communication with a "doormat," aggressive with a Mac truck, and assertive with a sage.

Caregivers might practice distinguishing between these three forms of communication, using examples from the group or from *Growing Wiser*. Scenarios might be drawn from a list of situations in which assertiveness may be helpful—for example, in refusing a request to borrow your car or your money; resisting sales pressure; asking a favor of someone; telling a person you are intimately involved with when he or she does or says something that bothers you; or continuing to converse with someone who disagrees with you. (These are drawn from an Assertion Inventory developed by Gambrill and Richey, 1975. The entire list can be found in the Fallcreek & Mettler, 1983). We have also used scenarios such as the following:

> Scenario: You have just seen the doctor regarding a skin problem your care receiver is experiencing. He has prescribed a cream you never heard of before. As you walk down the aisle away from the receptionist's desk, you realize that you do not understand how or when to use the cream. What do you do?

Participants can easily see themselves in this situation. Discussion can use a problem-solving focus as a vehicle for developing assertiveness skills. A possible assertive response might be:

> I quickly return to the receptionist and say, "I just realized that I need some additional information from Dr. Jones. If he is available, I would like to see him for just a minute." If the receptionist is surly, you may need to use the broken record technique in order to get her to do her job. If the doctor is already in with another patient, it would be aggressive to insist that he leave that patient to answer your question, so you say, "Since he is not available now, I would like to call him with my question. When would be a good time to reach him? Is it possible for him to give me a call? If so, would you give him the message?"

Other scenarios might focus on assertiveness in setting limits with the care receiver. For example, you just returned from an evening out with your friends. Your daughter was staying with your husband. You are very tired, but your husband wants to discuss the evening. After a 30-minute discussion, you are ready to go to bed, but he would like you to give him a bath. You bathed him earlier the same day.

A possible assertive response: "I love you very much, dear (you rub his shoulders thinking he may be asking for some physical contact). If I weren't feeling so tired, I would be glad to give you a bath. But tonight, I won't be able to do it. Let's plan on a bath tomorrow morning."

After the discussion of assertiveness, caregivers may benefit from a homework assignment. One assignment might ask them to make a list of statements they made that were (a) assertive, (b) passive, and (c) aggressive. This can stimulate interesting discussion in the following session.

Coping with Criticism Skills

Criticism can increase the stress experienced by caregivers (Spaid & Barusch, in press). Most often it comes from those closest to the caregiver, a son or daughter. Often those criticizing care deeply about the patient, but are not close enough to the daily situation to appreciate the demands placed on the caregiver.

Unfortunately, most people automatically feel anxious when they are criticized. As Manuel J. Smith pointed out in *When I Say No I Feel Guilty* (1987), we fail to distinguish between the truth and the fallacy in criticism. Usually, a critical remark is true in its description of our behavior. The fallacy that is implied by criticism is that the behavior is wrong or bad. For example, the comment "You've left Dad alone three times this week!" might be the first strike in a family battle if stated in a critical tone. Caregivers can learn to defuse the criticism by separating the truth—"Yes, I did leave him alone three times"—from the implied fallacy that this behavior is a sign of neglect or indifference. Three techniques—fogging, negative assertion, and negative inquiry—can be used to cope with criticism. These are drawn from *When I Say No I Feel Guilty* (Smith, 1987).

Communication Technique 2: Fogging

The goal of fogging is to serve as a fog bank for criticism. As Smith explained, "A fog bank is remarkable in some aspects. It is very persistent. We cannot see through it. It offers no resistance to our penetration. It does not fight back. . . . We can throw an object right through it, and it is unaffected. Inevitably, we give up trying to alter the persistent, independent, nonmanipulable fog and leave it alone" (1987, p. 104).

Fogging involves agreeing with that aspect of the criticism that is true. It requires listening to the content of the message without responding to its emotion-laden implications. The technique can be practiced in dyads, with one person being the critic and the other a "fogger." For example:

Critic:	"You sure look terrible today, don't you care at all about your appearance?"
Fogger:	"You're probably right, I'm not looking my best. I can see how you might think I didn't care about my looks."
Critic:	"If you dress that way other people will think you're a pig!"
Fogger:	"That could be true. It's possible they will think I'm a pig."
Critic:	"People who don't try to look their best usually are lazy and stupid."
Fogger:	"I suppose there could be a relationship between intelligence and appearance."

Fogging can be used when you begin to feel defensive, when a discussion could be side-tracked by criticism, when you need to stay focused, need to protect yourself emotionally, feel you are being baited, and when you want to stop a conversation. It enables you to accept criticism by calmly acknowledging to your critic the possibility that there is some truth in what he or she says, yet allows you to remain your own judge of what you do. You learn to receive criticism comfortably without becoming anxious or defensive, while giving no reward to those using manipulative criticism.

It is best not to use fogging to avoid an important discussion or to frustrate the other person. Sometimes negative feedback warrants a response. There are some risks in using fogging. It may discourage future feedback, both positive and negative, from the other person. It may keep you from listening or it may be used to avoid responsibility. It also tends to discount another person's point of view and conveys a message of indifference.

Communication Technique 3: Negative Assertion

Negative assertion can be used to cope with mistakes we have made without becoming upset in the face of criticism of these mistakes. Many of us react to mistakes by feeling guilty and anxious. This leads us to seek forgiveness or try to deny our mistakes. Instead, we can recognize our right to make mistakes (see Bill of Assertive Rights) and still be acceptable, even lovable human beings. Negative assertion is one technique in support of this position.

To use this technique, you simply agree with the criticism. You acknowledge your mistakes as if they were just that, no more or less. This, like fogging, can be practiced in dyads in which one person serves as critic and the other as negative asserter. The exercise will be most effective if the asserter first tells the critic about a real mistake he or she has made recently. For example:

Asserter:	Last week I forgot that my wife was allergic to strawberries. I gave them to her and she broke out in hives."
Critic:	"Boy! Mom looks terrible! You must have given her a food she's allergic to!"
Asserter:	"You're right, I did. What a forgetful thing to do! I feel terrible about it!"
Or:	
Critic:	Didn't you notice that 'Don't Walk' sign? You could have been killed!
Asserter:	You're right. I wasn't paying attention! What a dangerous thing to do!"

Negative assertion teaches you to accept your errors and faults (without having to apologize) by strongly and sympathetically agreeing with hostile or constructive criticisms of your negative qualities. You learn to look more comfortably at negatives in your own behavior or personality without feeling defensive and anxious or resorting to denial of real error, while at the same time reducing your critic's anger or hostility. It should only be used when you agree with the feedback. Negative assertion should not be used when you do not agree or when you are agreeing just to stop the communication.

The advantages of this technique are that it encourages ownership and responsibility and prevents defensiveness. It can also reduce anger of the other and assure him or her that you have understood the criticism. Its disadvantages are that it may be used to shut off communication and may be seen as an abrupt dismissal of the feedback.

A related skill, positive assertion, can be used to accept compliments. Using positive assertion you simply agree with a compliment: "Oh thank you! I like this dress too!" Or, if you aren't sure you agree, "Thank you for the compliment! I'm still not sure whether I like it or not. I'm glad you do!"

Communication Technique 4: Negative Inquiry

Negative inquiry involves active prompting of criticism in order to use the information (if helpful) or exhaust it (if manipulative) while helping your critic to be more assertive. Both fogging and negative assertion can reduce the amount of feedback you receive from people who do not like your behavior. Negative inquiry can be used to counteract this situation—to prompt the person who is complaining to provide more detailed information. If the complaint is legitimate this clarification may lead to problem solving.

For example:

Critic: "I don't like the way you're taking care of my father."

Inquirer: "What is it about my care that you don't like?"

Critic: "Well, you don't seem to respect his opinions."

Inquirer: "I'm not sure I understand. Which of his opinions do you feel I don't respect."

Critic: "The other day when I was visiting you wouldn't let him eat what he wanted."

Inquirer: "What was it that he wanted to eat?"

Critic: "He asked you for ice cream and you made him a sandwich instead."

Inquirer: "Oh! Now I see. You feel that I should have given him ice cream for lunch! Were you aware that he asks for ice cream at every meal? How often do you think I should give it to him?"

As in the example, negative inquiry can make caregivers more comfortable in viewing criticism as feedback. It can also assure the critic that his or her views are taken seriously.

Negative inquiry can be used whenever you want to open up communication or when feedback is important. It can also help when you are not sure how to interpret a comment. It should not be used to avoid expressing feelings by being rational or to negate or ridicule the feedback.

Managing Conflict

Like criticism, conflict can be an important source of stress for caregivers. Three techniques for managing conflict are presented here: broken record, workable compromise, and DESC scripting. Broken record and workable compromise were presented in *When I Say No I Feel Guilty* (Smith, 1987) and DESC scripting is drawn from Bower and Bower's *Asserting Yourself: A Practical Guide for Positive Change* (1984).

Communication Technique 5: Broken Record

The broken record technique is the most basic assertiveness skill. M. J. Smith said, "One of the most important aspects of being verbally assertive is to be persistent and to keep saying what you want over and over again without getting angry, irritated, or loud" (1987, p 74). This is the broken record technique. You calmly say what you want over and over again. This requires persistence. You do not have to rehearse arguments or angry feeling beforehand in order to be "up" for dealing with others, but you do have to know clearly what you want.

This technique can be especially effective in commercial and professional situations. Often clerks, public officials, bureaucrats, and secretaries have learned that saying no is easier than seriously considering a person's request. The broken record tests how many no they have at their disposal. It also makes it harder for them to say no than to take you seriously. For example:

Caregiver:	(talking to the physician's secretary) "I want the doctor to see my mother this week."
Secretary:	"The doctor is very busy, he doesn't have any open appointment until next week."

Caregiver:	"I understand that he is busy, and I want him to see my mother this week."
Secretary:	"You don't understand, the doctor's schedule is full this week."
Caregiver:	"I understand that his appointment schedule is full, and I want him to see my mother this week."
Secretary:	"I can't just let patients come in whenever they want to. It would be chaos around here!"
Caregiver:	"I understand how you feel, and I really want him to see my mother this week. Is there something we could do to make that easier for you?"
Secretary:	(Moving toward a solution.) "Well, are you willing to come in after 5:00?"
Caregiver:	Yes, if he will see my mother this week I will be glad to bring her in after 5:00" (a workable compromise).

This technique can be used to set the stage for the use of workable compromise described below. In order for the combination to be effective, it is important to be certain of what you want. The Broken Record should not be used when the point has been heard and responded to, when the other person becomes distressed by your use of it, or when you are not sure what you want.

Communication Technique 6: Workable Compromise

The workable compromise combines problem-solving and bargaining skills. The technique is most effective when the situation is seen as a problem shared by both parties involved in the conflict. This will engage the other person in your problem-solving efforts. In the above example, the caregiver made her need to see the doctor a shared concern and her success a foregone conclusion when she said, "What can we do to make this easier for you?" Similarly, when dealing with a reluctant bureaucrat a caregiver might say, "I know you want to do your job as well as possible. My mother needs this service. What can we do to help you meet her needs?"

Preparing for a compromise also involves deciding as early as possible what is and what is not negotiable. Self-respect, for example, is not. As M. J. Smith points out, "It is practical, whenever you feel that your self-respect is not in question, to offer a workable compromise to the other person" (1987, p. 84). You can always bargain for your material goals unless the compromise effects your personal feelings of self-respect. If the end goal involves a matter of your self worth, however, there can be no compromise. On the other hand, the caregiver in the above example may not care what time she has to bring her mother in, or how long she has to stay in the waiting room. Another example:

Caregiver:	"The therapist says that you can walk as far as the bathroom. want you to walk there by yourself."
Care Receiver:	"I'm not sure I can."
Caregiver:	"I understand that you don't feel confident and I want you walk there by yourself" (broken record).
Care Receiver:	"I'm afraid I might fall."
Caregiver:	"I understand, and I don't want you to fall. What can *we* do protect you and help you to walk there by yourself?" (established mutual problem-solving responsibility).
Care Receiver:	"I just don't know."
Caregiver:	"Are you willing to try something I propose?"
Care Receiver:	"Maybe."
Caregiver:	"Well, I need a commitment from you" (guarantees mutual effort).
Care Receiver:	"Oh, alright. What's your idea?"
Caregiver:	"Let's set a deadline. I want you to walk there by yourself, but it doesn't have to happen today. When do you think you'll be ready, and what do you think we'll need to do to get you ready? (Setting the stage for a compromise).

The advantage of workable compromise is that it engages both parties in an effort to solve the problem or conflict. It encourages respect for the other, and helps meet the caregiver's needs—at least to some extent. The technique brings the risk of giving up too soon, and may result in ignoring personal needs.

Communication Technique 7: DESC Scripting

DESC scripting can be used to resolve either short-term or long term conflicts. The technique is described in *Asserting Yourself: Practical Guide for Positive Change* by Sharon Bower and Gordon Bower (1984). The initials stand for the four steps involved in thi process of conflict resolution: describe, express, specify and consequences.

1. DESCRIBE the other person's behavior or the situation being reacted to specifically and objectively. In this step it is important to describe the behavior, not your reaction to it. For example, instead of starting with "You treat me like dirt," try, "You don't come home when you say you will."

2. EXPRESS your emotional reaction to the other person's behavior of the situation in a nonevaluative way. Instead of "You are such a jerk!" try, "This makes me feel like you don't love me."

3. SPECIFY one or two behavior changes you would like the person to make (ask for agreement). Mutuality is important in this step. It is important to ask for changes that are feasible. Do not set the person up to fail. Instead of "Would you just come home on time?" try, "If you are going to be late would you please call?"

4. Choose the positive CONSEQUENCES you are prepared to carry through. Tell the person what you can do for him or her if the agreement to change is kept (positive consequences).

As a caregiver is learning the DESC technique, it may be helpful to write a script for the interactions. In training, a worksheet might be used, with blanks for the caregiver to indicate how he or she will make each of the four steps. Then dyads might practice, giving each other feedback on the quality of delivery. With practice, caregivers will be able to use the technique without a script.

GRIEF AND LOSS EXERCISE: LETTING GO

Used in connection with a discussion of loss and grief, this exercise offers a powerful experience, increasing a caregiver's empathy for the dying person. Letting go sensitizes participants to the experience of losing everything that is part of dying. Leaders should be prepared for strong emotional reactions. This exercise should only be undertaken in an atmosphere of trust and support. Gentle music can be used to create a calm, soothing environment.

Instructions

First, take 10 slips of paper ("3 × 5" cards work well, and the number may vary). Then you will write ten different answers to one question; each answer will go on a separate sheet. The question is "Who are you?" Take a quiet moment to reflect, then put one answer on each sheet. Work fairly rapidly, without too much deliberation. No one will see your answers, just let them be spontaneous and meaningful.

[Allow 5-7 minutes for participants to fill in their answers.]

Now, reflect on the importance of each answer. Which answer is most central to your self-concept—to who you are? Which is least central? Organize the answers in order of importance. Number the cards, with the most important answer numbered "10," the least important, "1." Then arrange the cards in numerical order, with 1 on top and 10 on the bottom.

As J. Bugental pointed out,

> Nearly every ethical or religious tradition . . . has some concept of the importance of transcending or relinquishing the self. . . . We can easily see how this must tie into the interpretation of death as a letting go of much or all of that which has made up our lives. What these mystical traditions add is what others too have recognized: that this relinquishment may be the basis for a heightened vitality or meaningfulness in living. (p.157)

Now we will experience letting go of each of these aspects of your self-concept. We will start with the least important and work up to the more central aspects. We will focus on each card for a minute or so, to give you time to concentrate on the meaning of that aspect of your self-concept—how it has affected your life. Then, when I ring the bell, I want you to set aside the card and turn it over, letting go of that aspect of your identity. Consider how it feels. Give yourself some time to explore your reaction. Any feeling is okay. Sometimes people feel liberated by letting go, sometimes they feel sad. Do not evaluate your feelings, just notice them. When you are through, just relax and sit quietly until the bell rings again. Then, when the bell rings again, look at the next card in your pile. Repeat the process with this aspect of your identity. Consider what it has meant in your life and, when you are ready, let go. Spend a moment to reflect on how you feel.

[Leaders should allow about 2 minutes for each card.]

Choosing to Be. Some people find, once they have let go of each of their aspects that their ideas about what was most important have changed. Some parts that they initially thought were trivial turn out to be very hard to let go of. If this is true for you, renumber the cards, so that "10" indicates the aspect you are most eager to take back, and "1" indicates the one you are least eager to reassume. Use a different location for these numbers so you can later compare them with your earlier answers. Now, you will reassume each aspect of your self-concept, starting with those you are most eager to reclaim.

As J. Bugental explained,

> In so many regards, the ways in which we think of our own being seem to be imposed on us rather than chosen by us. If I think of the fact that I am a man or even a human being, that seems a product of biology not something of my own doing. Feeling that way about ourselves contributes to our feelings that we are powerless about what matters most in who we are. (p. 160)

If, instead of feeling "stuck" with certain aspects of our self-concept, we emphasize our power to choose, we will feel greater control of ourselves. Certainly we did not choose to be born human beings, men or women, but we can choose how we will interpret humanity, masculinity, and femininity. Now we will choose to reclaim each aspect of ourself. When you hear the bell, take the top card (number "10"). As you look at it, choose to take back that aspect of yourself, along with all it has meant to you. Give yourself a moment to experience how it feels to have it back. Then, when you hear the bell again, move on to the next card.

At the end of this exercise, participants need to take some time to talk about what they experienced. This is best accomplished in dyads, with plenty of time for sharing. Participants should choose a partner, someone they feel comfortable with, and take turns talking about their experiences. Then dyads should report back to the whole group on their discussions.

A BILL OF ASSERTIVE RIGHTS

I: You have the right to judge your own behavior, thoughts, and emotions, and to take the responsibility for their initiation and consequences upon yourself.

II: You have the right to offer no reasons or excuses for justifying your behavior.

III: You have the right to judge if you are responsible for finding solutions to other people's problems.

IV: You have the right to change your mind.

V: You have the right to make mistakes - and be responsible for them.

VI: You have the right to say, "I don't know."

VII: You have the right to be independent of the goodwill of others before coping with them.

VIII: You have the right to be illogical in making decisions.

IX: You have the right to say, "I don't understand."

X: You have the right to say, "I don't care." You have the right to say no without feeling guilty.

Source: Smith, M. (1975). The Bill of Assertive Rights. *When I say no I feel guilty,* pp. 185-186. Used by permission of Doubleday, a division of Bantam Doubleday Dell Publishing Group.

RESOURCES

Bugental, J. (1973). Confronting the existential meaning of my death through exercises *Interpersonal Development, 4,* 148-163.

Tubesing, N. L., & Tubesing, D. A. (Eds.). (1983). *A whole person handbook: Structured exercises in stress management.* Duluth, MN: Whole Person Press.

Visualization

Siegel, B. S. (1989). *Peace Love & Healing.* New York: Harper & Row.

Communication

Bower, S. A., & Bower, G. H. (1984). *Asserting yourself: A practical guide for positive change.* Reading, MA: Addison-Wesley.

APPENDIX C: Resources

General Books on Caregiver Support

Biegel, D. E. & Blum, A. (1990). *Aging and caregiving: Theory, research, and policy,* Newbury Park, CA: Sage.

Calder, A., & Watt, J. (1981). *I love you but you drive me crazy: A guide for caring relatives.* Vancouver, Canada: Forbez Publications. (2133 Quebec Street, Vancouver V57).

Fallcreek, S., & Mettler, M. (1983). A healthy old age: A sourcebook for health promotion with older adults (rev. ed.). *Journal of Gerontological Social Work, 6*(2/3).

Felder, L. (1990). *When a loved one is ill: How to take better care of your loved one, your family, and yourself.* New York: New American Library.

Hooyman, N. R., & Lustbader, W. (1986). *Taking care: Supporting older people and their families.* New York: Free Press.

Ideabook on caregiver support projects. Available for $6.50 from National Council on Aging, 600 Maryland Ave., S.W., Washington, DC 20024.

Kemper, D. W., Mettler, M., Guiffre, J., & Matzek, B. (1986). Growing wiser: The older person's guide to mental wellness. Boise, ID: Healthwise. (P.O. Box 1989, Boise, ID 83701; (208) 345-1161; cost: $10.00 + 2.50 for shipping)

Mace, N., & Rabins, P. (1982). *The 36-hour day.* Baltimore, MD: Johns Hopkins University Press (3400 N. Charles, Baltimore, MD 21218).

McDowell, F. (1980). *Managing the person with intellectual loss at home.* White Plains, NY: Burke Rehabilitation Institute (785 Mamoroneck Avenue, White Plains, NY 10605).

Montgomery, R. V. J. (Ed.). (1985). *Family seminars for caregiving: Helping families help.* Seattle: University of Washington Press (P.O. Box 50096, Seattle, WA 98145; (206)543-8870; cost: $50.00).

Pierslalla, C., & Heald, J. (1982). *Help for families of the aging.* Available from the National Support Center for Families of the Aging (P.O. Box 245, Swathmore, PA 19081).

Springer, D., & Brubaker, T. H. (1984). *Family caregivers and dependent elderly: Minimizing stress and maximizing independence.* Beverly Hills, CA: Sage.

Stokell, M., & Kennedy, B. (1985). *The senior citizen handbook: A self-help and resource guide.* Englewood Cliffs, NJ: Prentice-Hall.

Trocchio, J. (1981). *Home care of the elderly.* Boston: CBI Publishing (51 Sleeper Street, Boston, MA 02210).

Organizations

American Association of Retired Persons (AARP).

A membership organization for those over 50. A great source of information, AARP has offices in each region.

1909 K Street, N.W.
Washington, DC 20049
(800) 424-2277

Arthritis Foundation

A source of information. They operate support groups in some areas.

1314 Spring Street, N.W.
Atlanta, GA 30309
(404) 872-7100

National Hospice Organization

A good source of information.

1901 N. More St., Suite 901
Arlington, VA 22209
(703) 243-5900

Alzheimer's Disease and Related Disorders Association (ADRDA)

ADRDA has local chapters in many communities. An excellent source of information, they also run support groups.
(800) 621-0379; Illinois call: 800-572-6037

American Diabetes Association

Provides funds for research. A good source of information and will be starting a support group.

1660 Duke Street
Alexandria, VA 22314
(703) 549-1500
(800) 232-3472

American Heart Association

Provides funds for research. Also a source of pamphlets and weight control information.

7320 Greenville
Dallas, TX 75231
(214) 373-6300

American Cancer Society

Provides funds for cancer research, education, service and rehabilitation.

National office:
1599 Clifton Road, N.E. Atlanta, GA 30329
(404) 320-3333

These are just a few of the organizations that might be helpful to caregivers. For organizations that serve those with specific diseases, see Felder (1990).

INDEX

ABOUT THE AUTHOR

AMANDA SMITH BARUSCH is Associate Professor at the University of Utah Graduate School of Social Work. She chairs the gerontology emphasis and the human behavior sequence. Her teaching responsibilities are in the areas of human development, aging, and program administration. She has also served on the faculty of the University of Guam. She graduated from Reed College and completed both her MSW and PhD at the University of California, Berkeley. Amanda Smith Barusch has been working in the aging field for more than a decade. She has extensively investigated family care of the frail elderly, and the impact of services on family caregiving. Her work has appeared in *The Gerontologist, Journal of Gerontological Social Work, Journal of Social Service Research,* and *Journal of Sociology and Social Welfare;* and has been presented at numerous symposia. She has conducted research in the Western Pacific, Hong Kong, and China, studying intergenerational relationships, family dynamics, and the life-styles of elderly in areas experiencing rapid social change.